Foreword

I can wish this book every success, feeling completely confident that it will prove popular not only with examination candidates, but also with a wide range of clinicians. It is a fun book for those of us who do not have to face any more exams. The authors give enough information about each of the 60 patients to enable the reader to reach the correct diagnosis, but it is necessary for him to have his wits about him to pick up the important clues. The questions on investigations and treatment which follow each case presentation are quite testing even for someone working in gastroenterology. The answers and explanations given in the 60 commentaries are based on the latest advances in clinical and basic science. They will be most helpful for getting through the Membership as well as a painless update for the general physician.

Gastroenterology is a rapidly developing specialty, but it is still an integral part of general internal medicine and I was interested to note the number of patients who had few or trivial gastrointestinal symptoms. Many of the clinical problems discussed are conditions which can present to surgeons, so this book will be useful for Fellowship candidates as well as general surgeons, who will find added interest in the appendix on post-surgical syndromes. The subjects for the eight appendices are well chosen to deal with recent developments in the investigatory techniques and therapy of the specialty. The literary style throughout is light, often colloquial and remarkably uniform. I congratulate the young physician authors on having produced such an excellent, up-to-date and easy-to-read book.

R. B. McConnell
Liverpool

Other titles in preparation

Case Presentations in Chemical Pathology
Case Presentations in Endocrinology
Case Presentations in Neurology

Titles in the Series

Case Presentations in Paediatrics
Case Presentations in Heart Disease
Case Presentations in Renal Medicine

Case Presentations in Gastrointestinal Disease

W. D. W. Rees, MB BCh, MD, MRCP
Consultant Physician and Gastroenterologist, University of Manchester
Medical School, Hope Hospital, Salford

S. Hughes, MB ChB, MRCP
Senior Registrar in Gastroenterology, Royal Liverpool and Broadgreen
Hospitals, Liverpool

J. L. Shaffer, MB BS, MRCP
Lecturer and Honorary Senior Registrar in Gastroenterology and Clinical
Pharmacology, University of Manchester Medical School, Hope Hospital,
Salford

G. R. Barclay, MB ChB, MRCP
Research Fellow in Gastroenterology, University of Manchester Medical
School, Hope Hospital, Salford

Butterworths
London   Boston   Durban   Singapore   Sydney   Toronto   Wellington

First published, 1985

© **Butterworths & Co. (Publishers) Ltd, 1985**

British Library Cataloguing in Publication Data

Case presentations in gastrointestinal disease.
   1. Digestive organs — Diseases — Case studies
   I. Rees, W.D.W.
   616.3'09   RC801

   ISBN 0–407–00542–0

Library of Congress Cataloging in Publication Data

Case presentations in gastrointestinal disease.

   Includes bibliographies and index.
   1. Gastrointestinal system — Diseases — Case studies.
2. Gastrointestinal system — Diseases — Examinations
questions, etc. I. Rees, W. D. W. [DNLM: 1.
Gastroenterology — case studies. 2. Gastroenterology —
examination questions. WI 100 C337]
RC802.C37 1984   616.3'3'0076   84–15574
ISBN 0–407–00542–0

Photoset by Illustrated Arts Limited, Sutton, Surrey
Printed and bound by Cox & Wyman Ltd, Reading

Preface

Gastrointestinal problems are frequently encountered by the general practitioner, paediatrician, general physician and general surgeon. Butterworths' *Case Presentations in Gastrointestinal Disease* is one of a series of books designed to prepare candidates for higher professional examinations and provide useful and concise information for hospital based doctors and general practitioners. It is not a textbook of gastroenterology but provides a 'case-orientated' approach to common, as well as a number of less common, disorders involving the gastrointestinal tract, liver, biliary tree and pancreas.

The book consists of two sections. The first consists of 60 selected case histories covering a diversity of gastrointestinal diseases, followed by discussions on each of the cases. To assist candidates preparing for examinations, each history is followed by a series of questions which assess clinical acumen as well as factual knowledge. The answers to these questions precede the discussion of each case. The second section consists of eight concise reviews which highlight common investigative and management problems. Some of the major technological and therapeutic advances made in gastroenterology over the past decade are discussed and their value in patient management assessed.

In selecting these cases and review topics we have provided a blend of information which will assist examination candidates as well as practitioners dealing with gastrointestinal diseases. We are grateful to a number of colleagues at Hope Hospital, Salford, for providing some of the cases and to Mrs Julie Rostron who devoted many hours to preparing the manuscript.

The authors wish to dedicate this book to their wives Menna, Paula, Lindsey and Jean for their patience and support.

W. D. W. Rees
S. Hughes
J. L. Shaffer
G. R. Barclay

Contents

Foreword   v
Preface   vii

Part 1:   **1**

1   Case Presentations   1
2   Discussion of cases   47
3   Normal laboratory values   156

Part 2:   **159**

Reviews   159

   Management of peptic ulcer disease   159

   Post-surgical syndromes   163

   Investigation of jaundice   170

   Liver failure   174

   Assessment of pancreatic function   178

   Investigation of diarrhoea   184

   The diagnosis and management of Crohn's disease   190

   The assessment and management of nutritional deficiencies 195

Index of Cases   200

Part 1

1 Case presentations

Case 1

A 49-year-old electrician, with a 10 week history of anorexia and weight loss, developed acute abdominal pain. On admission to hospital he was found to be febrile, jaundiced, cachectic and had signs of peritonitis.

Investigations revealed a haemoglobin of 9.1 g/dl, white blood count of $12.8 \times 10^9/\ell$, ESR of 117 mm/hour, an albumin of 16 g/ℓ, raised hepatic enzymes (alkaline phosphatase of 430 IU/ℓ and AST of 215 IU/ℓ) and a prolonged prothrombin time (17 seconds versus a control time of 13 seconds). Emergency laparotomy revealed a leaking sigmoid colon abscess, but, apart from hepatomegaly, the liver and biliary tree appeared normal. A sigmoid colectomy was performed, but following surgery he developed signs of right lower lobe consolidation with rigors and his liver function tests deteriorated. A wedge liver biopsy obtained at laparotomy showed non-specific hepatitis and cultures of his blood and sputum were persistently negative. An ultrasound scan of the liver and biliary tree demonstrated multiple hypoechoic lesions in the right hepatic lobe and these were confirmed by CT scanning.

Questions

1. What is the most likely cause of his liver disease?
2. What diagnostic test would confirm the nature of this disease?

Case 2

A 63-year-old woman was admitted with a 10 day history of diarrhoea and abdominal swelling. She was passing 8 liquid stools a day without blood or mucus. Prior to her illness she had been consti-pated for years, but had no other abdominal symptoms. In the past she had received radioactive phosphorus (^{32}P) for polycythaemia rubra vera. Two months before admission she had developed anaemia and bruising secondary to acute myeloid leukaemia. This was treated by combination cytotoxic chemotherapy and she developed a septicaemia which was treated by intravenous genta-micin, lincomycin and later flucloxacillin. After a further course of chemotherapy she was discharged on septrin, allopurinol and fungilin. Five days later she developed diarrhoea.

On examination she was pyrexial (temperature 38°C), had ascites and marked peripheral oedema. Rectal examination revealed a nodular mucosa and the absence of faeces. At sigmoidoscopy the mucosa had a reddened polypoid appearance with white exudate. Blood tests revealed a haemoglobin of 9.8 g/dl, white cell count of $1.4 \times 10^9/\ell$, serum albumin of 28 g/ℓ, and normal liver enzymes. Serum potassium was 2.9 mmol/ℓ and blood urea 17.0 mmol/ℓ.

Questions

1. What is the most likely diagnosis?
2. What three tests should be done to confirm the diagnosis?
3. What treatment should be given?

Case 3

A 30-year-old housewife presented with a 4 year history of diarrhoea with mucus, accompanied by slight weight loss. In the past she had tended to be constipated. Sigmoidoscopy showed a reddened mucosa and a rectal biopsy mild non-specific inflamma-tion. Barium enema was normal. Treatment with sulphasalazine was unsuccessful, but she improved after a course of oral steroids.

However, the response was temporary and she developed further diarrhoea and episodes of left iliac fossa pain. In addition she had become very depressed. Despite relatively limited disease she was treated with a total colectomy and ileostomy. Histology showed some thinning of the rectal mucosa and minimal inflammation without ulceration. She improved initially but subsequently developed ileostomy diarrhoea (up to 5 ℓ/day). Physical examination and barium meal and follow-through were normal at this time. She had three episodes during which the serum potassium fell (as low as 1.9 mmol/ℓ) and her plasma pH rose to 7.7 (bicarbonate 38 mmol/ℓ). These responded to appropriate intravenous supplements. She was referred for further investigations.

Questions

1. What three diagnoses should be considered?
2. Name three helpful investigations.

Case 4

A 34-year-old man was admitted urgently by his general practitioner following 3 hours of severe central abdominal colic radiating into the back. The pain was associated with anorexia and nausea, but there was no vomiting or alteration in bowel habit. Over the previous 2 years he had experienced similar, although less severe pain, lasting up to 3 days and accompanied by loose pale motions. He drank 2 pints of beer and smoked 20 cigarettes per day. Investigations at another hospital had apparently failed to arrive at a diagnosis.

On examination, the patient was in severe pain, pale, sweaty, and had brownish pigmentation on his face, lips, trunk and hands. His pulse was 106/min and blood pressure 90/60 mmHg. His abdomen was extremely tender with rebound tenderness, and there was a mass in the right iliac fossa. Bowel sounds were absent and his rectum was empty. On admission to a local hospital his haemoglobin was 9 g/dl, MCH 24 pg, MCHC 20 g/dl, white cell count 13.0 × 10^9/ℓ, and electrolytes were normal. Plain abdominal X-ray showed no abnormality.

Questions

1. Name two possible diagnoses and state which is more likely.
2. What further information from the history would be helpful in making this diagnosis?
3. List three complications of this condition?

Case 5

A 47-year-old man presented with a 5 year history of intermittent epigastric discomfort, waterbrash and vomiting. The symptoms were initially relieved by food and antacids but had become progressively worse and more persistent. There was no family history of peptic ulcer disease and no past medical history of relevance. Physical examination revealed epigastric tenderness only and full blood count, urea and electrolytes and liver function tests were normal. Upper gastrointestinal endoscopy demonstrated the presence of duodenal ulcer with marked duodenitis and he was instructed to stop smoking and was prescribed a 6 week course of cimetidine (400 mg b.d.). He remained symptomatic, and 2 months later was prescribed a course of colloidal bismuth. After a further 6 week period repeat endoscopy showed an active duodenal ulcer with duodenitis. A proximal gastric vagotomy was therefore performed, but 2 months after operation he developed severe epigastric pain and vomited blood stained material. Investigations revealed a haemoglobin of 10.2 g/dl, a microcytic, hypochromic blood film and serum calcium of 2.85 mmol/ℓ. Upper gastrointestinal endoscopy showed recurrence of a duodenal ulcer and a truncal vagotomy with antrectomy was performed. During the post-operative period the patient developed intractable vomiting necessitating parenteral nutrition and continuous nasogastric aspiration.

Questions

1. What is the most likely diagnosis?
2. Name two investigations that would confirm the diagnosis.
3. List two further tests that would be useful in the further management of this condition.
4. What is the significance of the hypercalcaemia?

Case 6

A 60-year-old woman presented to her general practitioner with a 6 month history of frequent heartburn, epigastric pain and acid reflux. Her symptoms were particularly troublesome in bed at night, and on several occasions she had woken up with chest tightness, coughing and wheezing, lasting up to 2 hours. She had no dysphagia or vomiting and her weight had increased by 3 kg in the preceding 4 months. Previously she had been fairly fit except for incontinence of urine, for which she had been prescribed emepronium bromide (2 tablets t.d.s), and intermittent ankle oedema. She was a widow living alone and worked as a part-time cleaner. Several times a week she attended a social club and drank 5 or 6 whiskies on each occasion. In addition, she smoked 20 cigarettes a day.

On examination, she was obese but otherwise fit. There was no ankle oedema or abdominal abnormalities. Routine blood count, electrolytes and liver function tests were normal. Barium meal showed a small sliding hiatus hernia with free reflux, and gastroscopy at a local hospital revealed moderate oesophagitis but no stricture formation.

Questions

1. What five factors mentioned in the case history may be relevant to her oesophagitis?
2. What is the significance of her nocturnal respiratory problems?
3. Which infective agents cause oesophagitis?

Case 7

A 22-year-old hairdresser presented with a 4 week history of diarrhoea (without bleeding), nausea, anorexia and 3 kg weight loss. The symptoms started 4 weeks after a course of ampicillin for urinary tract infection. Examination was normal as were the initial investigations (full blood count and stool culture). A diagnosis of post antibiotic diarrhoea was made and she was discharged when her symptoms had resolved. She presented 6 weeks later with a recurrence of diarrhoea accompanied by peri-umbilical pain. In addition she complained of anorexia, further weight loss, intermittent vomiting and marked lethargy. She also admitted to recent oral aphthous ulcers, backache and 2 days before admission had noticed some red spots on her legs. For the past 6 years she had been to Spain, Italy and Greece for summer holidays.

On examination she looked unwell, had a temperature of 38.4°C and conjunctival injection of her right eye. Several 1–2 cm tender, papular lesions were present on the extensor surface of her knees and elbows. Abdominal examination revealed left sided tenderness, no masses or visceromegaly, and normal bowel sounds. Her perineum was healthy but two skin tags were noted around the anal margin. Investigations revealed a haemoglobin of 12.9 g/dl, WBC $9 \times 10^9/\ell$, ESR 100 mm/hour, normal albumin, liver function tests and electrolytes.

Questions

1. What is the most likely diagnosis?
2. What is the nature of her skin lesions?
3. List three investigations that would help confirm the diagnosis?

Case 8

A 58-year-old woman presented to her general practitioner with a 6 month history of suprasternal dysphagia to solid food, but not liquids. She had no heartburn or anorexia, but had lost 6 kg in weight. She also complained of tiredness, exertional dyspnoea, gritty eyes and a dry mouth. In the past she had been diagnosed as having small bowel Crohn's disease and seronegative arthropathy, for which she had taken Naproxen and prednisolone for many years.

On examination she was pale, had angular stomatitis and brittle, spoon-shaped nails. There was no lymphadenopathy and her thyroid was not enlarged. No significant abdominal abnormality was present. Haemoglobin was 8.6 g/dl and MCH 22.9 pg, with hypochromia and microcytosis on the blood film. Serum iron was $2 \mu mol/\ell$, total iron binding capacity $52 \mu mol/\ell$, and albumin 28 g/ℓ. An upper intestinal endoscopy was normal.

Questions

1. What is the most likely cause of the dysphagia?
2. Name one investigation that would confirm the diagnosis.
3. What is the most likely explanation of the iron and TIBC results?
4. What other syndrome does this patient have, and how can it be confirmed?

Case 9

An 85-year-old woman was admitted to hospital with a 2 day history of colicky peri-umbilical pain, abdominal distension and absolute constipation. Three days prior to this episode she had experienced right upper quadrant discomfort and rigors lasting 36 hours but this subsided without specific therapy. She had a long history of flatulent dyspepsia and a duodenal ulcer was diagnosed by her general practitioner at the age of 63 years. She was prescribed an 'ulcer diet' and antacids and her symptoms had been reasonably well controlled since. On examination, she appeared dehydrated, had a tachycardia of 120/min and blood pressure of 90/50 mmHg. Her abdomen appeared distended and she was tender in the right hypochondrium. Visible peristalsis was present in the peri-umbilical region and she had hyperactive bowel sounds. Hernial orifices were intact, there were no abdominal scars, and rectal examination revealed no faecal material.

Investigations showed a haemoglobin of 16 g/dl, WBC of $16.0 \times 10^9/\ell$, urea of 13.4 mmol/ℓ, bilirubin of 32 μmol/ℓ, alkaline phosphatase of 320 UI/ℓ and gamma GT of 430 IU/ℓ. Plain abdominal X-rays revealed dilated loops of small bowel with numerous fluid levels, a small opacity in the right iliac fossa and an 'abnormal gas pattern' in the right upper quadrant. She was therefore given intravenous fluids and prepared for laparotomy.

Questions

1. What is the diagnosis?
2. List the three most common causes of intestinal obstruction in an elderly person living in the UK.
3. What further investigations would you perform to establish the diagnosis in the above patient?

Case 10

A 31-year-old woman was admitted via the Casualty Department because of recent onset of exertional dyspnoea. Prior to admission she had noticed black stools for 24 hours but denied dyspepsia, bowel disturbance or previous bleeding. At the age of 16 years she had been noted to have Turner's syndrome on the basis of physical appearance, primary amenorrhoea and chromosomal studies. She had a long psychiatric history of depression, withdrawal and anti-social behaviour and was on diazepam, amitriptyline and depot injections of a phenothiazine drug.

Clinical examination revealed pallor and the features of Turner's syndrome. Abdominal examination was normal but rectal examination confirmed melaena. Investigations revealed a haemoglobin of 5.6 g/dl with a microcytic, hypochromic blood film. Serum iron was 3 mmol/ℓ and TIBC 84 mmol/ℓ. Barium meal and gastroscopy showed no lesion in the upper GI tract and barium enema was normal. After transfusion she remained well for 2 weeks but then bled again, her haemoglobin falling to 7 g/dl. Colonoscopy was performed and examination to the caecal pole revealed no abnormality. Over a period of 4 weeks she had several other self-limiting episodes of melaena.

Questions

1. What is the significance of her initial haematological results?
2. What three further investigations should be carried out to identify the cause of her bleeding?
3. How could her Turner's syndrome be related to the present problem?

Case 11

A 14-year-old school girl with personality problems, poor concentration in her class, outbreaks of temper tantrums and auditory hallucinations was referred to a psychiatrist. On questioning her parents a 3 year history was obtained of progressive dysarthria, tremor and more recently, clumsy movements of the hands and feet. Her schoolwork had also markedly deteriorated. She had a past history of migraine and periodic attacks of feeling faint and dizzy, sometimes passing out.

On examination she looked well and the abnormal findings were confined to the CNS. She had spastic paraparesis, a spastic dysarthria and early flexural contracture of both hands (left greater than right). Power was only slightly decreased and sensation was normal. Investigations revealed a haemoglobin of 12.7 g/dl, MCV 80 fl, WBC 6.2 × 10⁹/ℓ with a normal differential and ESR 2 mm/hour. Urea and electrolytes were normal, albumin 36 g/ℓ, globulin 31 g/ℓ, bilirubin 7 μmol/ℓ, ALT 90 IU/ℓ, AST 89 IU/ℓ, gamma GT 7 IU/ℓ and alkaline phosphatase 161 IU/ℓ. Skull and chest X-ray were normal and 24 hour urine showed mild generalized amino-aciduria. The CSF was normal in appearance and on microscopy.

Questions

1. What diagnosis should be considered?
2. What clinical test should be performed?
3. Name four helpful investigations.

Case 12

A 49 year-old man presented with a 27 year history of lower substernal 'fullness' and vomiting of undigested food. The symptoms occurred after consumption of liquids or solids, and were unaffected by the temperature of ingested material. Alcohol and fizzy drinks had no effect on his symptoms. He denied chest pain and was not prone to heartburn. Initially the symptoms were intermittent and controlled by chewing food well and drinking plenty of liquid. However, his symptoms became progressively worse and during the preceding 2 years vomiting was extremely troublesome. In addition he had begun to wake up at night with coughing and wheezing. His appetite was maintained and he had not lost weight. In the past, while serving in the army, he travelled to Korea, Greece and the United States of America. Family history revealed that his brother had similar symptoms. On examination, he looked well and was slightly overweight. Respiratory, cardiovascular, and abdominal examinations were normal. Routine blood tests and ECG showed no abnormality but a chest X-ray showed a widened mediastinum.

Questions

1. What is the most likely diagnosis?
2. What three further investigations would you request?
3. Name two methods of treating this condition.

Case 13

A 28 year-old teacher presented with a 3 year history of intermittent vomiting, diarrhoea with faecal incontinence and syncopal attacks. Six months earlier a cholecystectomy was performed because of cholesterosis and diverticula of the gall bladder. She had no other relevant past medical history. Family history revealed that her father had died from heart block at the age of 47 years. On examination, she appeared thin and had evidence of postural hypotension (blood pressure lying 110/70 mmHg, standing 70/30 mmHg). Abdominal examination was normal but rectal examination revealed poor anal sphincter tone and the presence of watery stools. She had slight irregularity of both pupils and a slow light reflex. Dorsiflexion of both feet was weak, cutaneous sensation was diminished below both knees and ankle jerks absent.

Investigations revealed a normal full blood count, ESR, fasting glucose, urea and electrolytes, liver function tests and chest X-ray. Urinalysis and stool cultures revealed no abnormality. Stool osmolality was 594 mosmol/kg and the sodium and potassium concentrations 80 and 87 mmol/ℓ respectively. Faecal fat output was 34 mmol/ day and 5 hour urinary xylose excretion 4% of a 5 g oral dose. Barium meal and follow through revealed flocculation and segmentation of the barium.

Questions

1. What is the most likely diagnosis and state one investigation that would confirm this?
2. What is the mechanism of steatorrhoea in this disorder and list two investigations that would help establish the cause of the fat malabsorption?

Case 14

The three-year-old son of an Irish tinker was admitted with a 24 hour history of colicky central abdominal pain. The family travelled from place to place living in a caravan. Six months previously, in another city, the boy had been treated by a general practitioner for 'mild pneumonia'. For 3 weeks he had complained of intermittent vague abdominal pains, occasional vomiting and several episodes of mild diarrhoea, without blood or mucus. His appetite was very good but despite this he was losing weight. The parents had noticed worms in his stools on several occasions during the week prior to admission.

On examination, the boy was vomiting and in pain. The abdomen was distended with gas and there was tenderness and guarding in both iliac fossae. Bowel sounds were increased and rectal examination revealed an empty rectum. The hernial orifices were intact and the child's temperature was 37.8°C. Full blood count showed a normal haemoglobin and the white cell count was $10 \times 10^9/\ell$. Differential white cell count revealed 67% polymorphs, 25% lymphocytes and 8% eosinophils. Urea and electrolytes and liver function tests were normal. Straight X-ray of the abdomen showed dilated loops of small bowel with fluid levels.

Questions

1. What is the most likely diagnosis?
2. What is the likely site of the obstruction and what is the procedure of choice at laparotomy?
3. What treatment should he receive after surgery?

Case 15

A 79-year-old baker presented with a 5 year history of left iliac fossa pain, and intermittent rectal bleeding for 3 months. The pain was aching in nature, present on most days and radiated into the groin. It usually lasted 1–2 hours but on two occasions had persisted for several days and was accompanied by a high fever. The rectal bleeding consisted of bright red blood mixed with faeces with occasional staining of the toilet paper. For many years he had defaecated only 1–2 times per week, passing small hard faeces, but was otherwise well. There was a family history of coronary artery disease and diabetes. He drank little alcohol, smoked 20 cigarettes per day and took no drugs. On examination he appeared fit and well. There was a systolic murmur audible at the left sternal edge, radiating into the aortic area and carotids. In the abdomen there was a palpable, slightly tender descending colon and rectal examination with protoscopy revealed haemorrhoids. Sigmoidoscopy was otherwise normal to 13 cms. Haemoglobin was 11.1 g/dl, white cell count $11 \times 10^9/\ell$ with 87% neutrophils, 8% lymphocytes, 4% monocytes and 1% basophils. ESR was 28 mm/hour and urea, electrolytes and liver function tests were normal. Plain X-ray of the abdomen was also normal.

Questions

1. What is the most likely diagnosis?
2. Name four other possible causes for his rectal bleeding.
3. What two further investigations are indicated?
4. What explains his more severe pain and fever?

Case 16

A 22-year-old man presented with a 5 year history of intermittent upper abdominal pain, radiating to the back, lasting 4 hours at a time, and occuring several times per week. No precipitating factors were identified and only analgesics provided relief. It was associated with frequent, pale, loose motions, which were difficult to flush and weight loss of 25 kg despite a good appetite. In the preceding months he had developed thirst and polyuria and since childhood had been prone to recurrent chest infections. He smoked 20 cigarettes per day, but did not drink excess alcohol.

On examination he was thin and centrally cyanosed but had no finger clubbing or jaundice. He was tender in the epigastrium and his chest was hyperinflated, with widespread expiratory rhonchi. Blood count, urea, electrolytes, albumin, calcium, and liver function tests were normal. The blood glucose was 37.0 mmol/ℓ, and serum amylase 99 IU/ℓ. Faecal fat was 57.5 mmol/day. The FEV_1 was 1.05 ℓ, FVC 2.13 ℓ (ratio 49%), peak expiratory flow rate 100 ℓ/min and transfer factor 20.66 ml/min/mmHg (predicted normal 82.1).

Questions

1. What is the most likely cause of his gastrointestinal symptoms?
2. What two non-invasive investigations would confirm this?
3. What two conditions could produce both his gastrointestinal and pulmonary symptoms, and how may these be diagnosed?
4. Outline the three main aims of treatment in this patient?

Case 17

A 26-year-old Indian presented with a 4 month history of malaise, anorexia, weight loss of 6 kg and night sweats. He had been resident in the UK for 8 years but had spent a short holiday in India 10 months before the onset of symptoms. There was no history of contact with infectious disease and he had no past history of relevance. Further questioning revealed he had intermittent discomfort in the right iliac fossa and abdominal distension, but no change in bowel habit. Physical examination demonstrated a pyrexia of 38.5°C, some generalized wasting, mild tenderness in the right iliac fossa and a palpable spleen (1cm below costal margin). Routine investigations showed a normal haemoglobin and white blood count, ESR of 78 mm/hour, normal fasting glucose, urea, electrolytes and liver function tests. Urinalysis and urine microscopy were normal as were plain X-rays of the chest and abdomen. No acid fast bacilli were detected in gastric lavage samples or early morning urine specimens and both liver biopsy and bone marrow aspiration were normal on histological and bacteriological examinations. A Mantoux test was negative (1 in 10 000) and a thick blood film revealed no evidence of parasites. CT scan of the abdomen was normal apart from confirming splenomegaly. A barium meal and follow through examination was performed and showed an abnormal segment of terminal ileum with deformity of the caecal pole.

14

Questions

1. What are the three most likely diagnoses?
2. List three ways in which these diagnoses may be distinguished.
3. What therapeutic agents are effective in treating these three diseases?

Case 18

A 59-year-old woman attended the outpatient clinic complaining of incomplete rectal evacuation and occasional soiling. For 7 years she had been constipated, passing small pellety stools with mucus and a little blood. Five years previously she had attended her general practitioner because of similar symptoms and treatment with bran had produced some improvement. She was taking Moduretic and a non-steroidal anti-inflammatory drug for 'rheumatism'.

Physical examination revealed no abnormality but at sigmoido-scopy there was copious mucus present in the rectum and at 6 cm there was a patch of reddened friable mucosa 3 cm across, on the left lateral wall of the rectum. Biopsy of the abnormal area revealed infiltration of an intact mucosa by acute inflammatory cells and fibrosis in the lamina propria extending up between the mucosal crypts. Smooth muscle fibres were also seen in the sub-mucosa. Barium enema was normal as was her full blood count, ESR and biochemical profile.

Questions

1. What is the diagnosis?
2. What aetiological factors have been incriminated in this condition?
3. How can this disorder be treated?

Case 19

A 50-year-old home help presented to her general practitioner with a 12 month history of generalized pruritis which was worse at night and during hot weather. There was no history of jaundice, pale stools or dark urine. The patient was a known asthmatic and had a past history of hay fever. There was no weight loss, anorexia or change in bowel habit. She was married with three teenage sons, one of whom had asthma and eczema, and the family had a cat, a dog and a budgerigar. Her current medication consisted of a cromogly-cate inhaler only. On examination she was tanned, had scratch marks on her arms and legs, and xanthomata around the eyelids. Her abdomen was slightly distended but there was no organome-galy. The remainder of the examination was normal. Investigations revealed a haemoglobin of 13 g/dl; WBC 9 × $10^9/\ell$, (60% neutro-phils, 32% lymphocytes, 5% monocytes, 2% basophils, 1% eosinophils); ESR 36 mm/hour; albumin 30 g/ℓ; globulin 40 g/ℓ; bilirubin 18 μmol/ℓ; AST 63 IU/ℓ; ALT 109 IU/ℓ; alkaline phos-phatase 960 IU/ℓ; and gamma GT 110 IU/ℓ.

Questions

1. What is the diagnosis?
2. Name four helpful investigations.
3. What is the best therapy for her pruritis?
4. What is the most useful indicator of her prognosis?

Case 20

A 65-year-old man presented with a 12 hour history of severe colicky left sided abdominal pain. A few hours after the onset of pain he developed vomiting and diarrhoea, with mucus and blood. Dur-ing the preceding three months he had experienced similar but less severe attacks of abdominal pain, especially after meals. His only other problem was angina, of 5 years duration, which was adequately controlled with Nifedipine and he denied taking other drugs.

On examination his temperature was 38°C and he looked pale. Pulse rate was 108/min and the blood pressure 105/50 mmHg. Pulses in both feet were absent, but the skin was healthy. His abdomen was tender with guarding over the left side, there were no palpable masses or abdominal bruit, and bowel sounds were present. Rectal examination showed the presence of dark red blood only. Investiga-tions revealed a white cell count of 15.6 × $10^9/\ell$, haemoglobin 11.2 g/dl, and normal urea, electrolytes, albumin, and plain abdomi-nal X-ray.

Questions

1. List six possible diagnoses and state which is most likely.
2. What three investigations would be most helpful in identifying the cause?
3. Name two complications of the most likely diagnosis.

Case 21

A 35-year-old Iranian student developed attacks of watery diarrhoea 3 days after returning from holiday on the west coast of Africa. He had watery stools 6 – 8 times per day, accompanied by blood and mucus. Treatment with anti-diarrhoeal agents failed and he was referred to the local hospital for further assessment. At this time he appeared well and the diarrhoea had markedly improved. Examination was normal apart from mild left iliac fossa discomfort. Rectal examination revealed semi-formed faecal material and sigmoidoscopy showed oedema of the rectal mucosa. The patient subsequently brought a stool sample to the hospital and microscopy demonstrated numerous red and white blood cells but no evidence of parasitic infestation. Culture of this sample revealed no pathogenic bacteria and mild colitis was diagnosed. He was treated with loperamide, Salazopyrine (1 g b.d.) and a topical steroid preparation. Ten days later he required urgent admission because of malaise, fever, abdominal cramps and recurrence of watery diarrhoea. These symptoms had developed gradually over 10 days and he passed 6 – 8 watery stools containing moderate amounts of fresh blood. On examination he appeared ill, had a fever of 38.5°C, tachycardia of 110/min and marked tenderness over the iliac fossae and epigastrium. There was no guarding or rigidity and bowel sounds were present. Sigmoidoscopy revealed the presence of fluid stools, mucus and blood and the mucosa was friable with contact bleeding.

Questions

1. What is the most likely diagnosis?
2. What are the two best methods of establishing this diagnosis?
3. What four drugs are used to treat this condition?

Case 22

A 35-year-old woman was admitted as an emergency with small bowel obstruction. Six months prior to admission she had intermittent diarrhoea and colicky abdominal pain. At laparotomy a strictured area in the terminal ileum was noted to be the site of obstruction and a 40 cm segment of ileum was resected. The remaining small bowel and colon appeared normal and histology revealed transmural inflammation with non-caseating granulomata consistent with Crohn's disease. She left hospital 14 days after surgery.

Six months post-operatively she attended the outpatient department complaining of watery diarrhoea. Although free of pain since the operation she passed 3 or 4 watery stools a day, usually immediately after breakfast. She occasionally passed a more formed stool later in the day. Her weight was steady and she was on no medication. Apart from a well healed laparotomy scar clinical examination was negative. Haemoglobin was 11.5 g/dl with normal indices. Serum B_{12} was 200 ng/ml and serum folate was 10.0 $\mu g/\ell$. Urea and electrolytes and liver function tests were normal. Barium follow-through and barium enema examinations showed no abnormality.

Questions

1. What is the most likely cause of the post-operative diarrhoea?
2. What two investigations may be helpful?
3. How should she be treated?
4. What replacement therapy may she require?

Case 23

A 60-year-old Irish housewife had a long history of ill health with 'anaemia' and 'bone pains' and a number of operations had been performed in the past to correct valgus deformities of her knees. Recent X-rays of her hips and knees showed a reduction in bone density, a fissure fracture of the right patella and marked bowing of the pelvic bones and femora. She also complained of diarrhoea, 4 times a day, for several years; weight loss of 8 Kg and leg cramps with tingling of her face and hands. There was a past history of pulmonary tuberculosis treated with streptomycin, para-amino salicylic acid and isoniazid. She had been married for 30 years and was born in Dublin. Alcohol consumption was moderate and she smoked 25 cigarettes per day. The drug history included paracetamol, ibuprofen and a herbal 'tonic'. Examination revealed short stature (height 150 cms), pallor, angular stomatitis and widespread bony tenderness with proximal muscle weakness. Abdominal examination was normal. Investigations showed a haemoglobin of 9.9 g/dl and MCV of 102 fl. Blood film showed target cells, macrocytes and Howell–Jolly bodies. Albumin was 24 g/ℓ; globulin 34 g/ℓ; corrected calcium 1.6 mmol/ℓ; magnesium 0.36 mmol/ℓ; bilirubin 11 μmol/ℓ; alkaline phosphatase 200 IU/ℓ; AST 20 IU/ℓ; ALT 19 IU/ℓ and gamma GT 14 IU/ℓ. Faecal fat output was 28 mmol/day (3 day collection).

Questions

1. What is the most likely diagnosis?
2. How may this be confirmed?
3. State two explanations for the abnormal haematological results?

Case 24

A 26-year-old woman presented to casualty with a sudden onset of severe upper abdominal pain of 1 hour's duration. Prior to this she had been well. There was no history of trauma, she smoked 20 cigarettes per day, but did not drink alcohol. She was on no medication other than the contraceptive pill, which she had taken for 6 years without problems.

On examination she was pale with cold clammy peripheries. Her pulse was 120/min and blood pressure 80/40 mmHg. The abdomen was extremely tender with guarding in the right hypochondrium and local rebound tenderness over a palpable right hepatic lobe. A systolic bruit was heard in this area. Bowel sounds were present and normal.

Haemoglobin was 9.1 g/dl, but urea, electrolytes, liver function tests, and amylase were normal. Plain abdominal X-ray showed no free air or dilated loops of bowel.

Questions

1. What is the most likely diagnosis?
2. What two investigations will confirm the diagnosis?

Case 25

A 25-year-old telephonist presented to her general practitioner with a 2 year history of recurrent, left upper quadrant, stabbing pain radiating into the back. She had always been constipated but 6 months before the onset of pain had an episode of watery diarrhoea lasting 5 days, whilst on holiday in Spain. Since then she had episodes of diarrhoea alternating with longer periods of constipation. On occasions her stools contained 'worm-like' structures but she had never noticed rectal bleeding. She complained of malaise, palpitations and frequency of micturition but her appetite was good and weight steady. Five years previously she had an appendicectomy but denied other illnesses or operations. On examination she appeared well, had a fine tremor of both hands and cold sweaty palms. Abdominal palpation revealed tenderness in the epigastrium, left upper quadrant and left iliac fossa. The remainder of the examination was normal including a digital examination of the rectum. Investigations revealed a normal full blood count, ESR, electrolytes and liver function tests. An MSU was normal on microscopy and negative for pathogens, ECG revealed sinus rhythm with normal complexes, and thyroid function was normal.

Questions

1. List three possible diagnoses.
2. What would be the three most useful investigations to help differentiate between these disorders?
3. What three therapeutic measures may improve this patient's symptoms?

Case 26

A 60-year-old decorator was admitted for investigation of chronic diarrhoea. During World War II he had been a prisoner of war in various camps in South East Asia and during this period (1941 to 1945) had been severely malnourished with a body weight of 32 Kg. During his captivity he had many episodes of profuse bloody diarrhoea, malaria and 'wet' Beri Beri. Towards the end of his captivity he developed progressive loss of vision and a scaly rash around his neck. Following his release he gained weight and recovered his sight but slight oedema of the legs persisted. His stools although normal before the war were never normal afterwards. He passed pale, offensive motions which were difficult to flush and over the years stool frequency gradually increased to 5 times a day. Despite this he felt perfectly well and his weight was steady. He worked normally, and it was only through the insistence of his wife that he attended the out-patient clinic. At presentation he was on no regular medication and drank little alcohol.

Physical examination revealed a well nourished man with slight oedema of the lower legs and ankles. Ward testing of the urine revealed ¼% glycosuria. Full blood count and biochemical profile were normal but barium meal and follow-through showed a non-specific malabsorption pattern. Three day faecal fat estimation confirmed steatorrhoea, with fat excretion of 71.5 mmol/day. Jejunal biopsy was normal.

Questions

1. What is the most likely cause of his malabsorption?
2. What was the likely cause of his blindness?
3. What was the significance of the rash around his neck?

Case 27

A 57-year-old engineer presented to the outpatient clinic with a 6 week history of polyuria, polydipsia and 13 Kg weight loss. In addition he complained of pain and discomfort in his right knee and both ankles, and a fortnight before admission had become impotent. There was a past history of pleurisy and herpes zoster affecting the left side of his chest. His wife and three teenage daughters had all been well. He was a non-smoker and drank 7–8 pints of beer per week. Examination revealed diminution of body hair, testicular atrophy and a 6 cm enlarged, smooth liver. There was discomfort on moving both ankles and right knee associated with crepitus, but there was no evidence of active synovitis. Urine investigation revealed the presence of glycosuria. Haemoglobin was 14.4 g/ℓ; MCV 101 fl; white count 6.3 × 10^9/ℓ; platelets count 144 × 10^9/ℓ; ESR 20 mm/hour; and prothrombin time 14 seconds (control 13 seconds). Urea and electrolytes were normal, albumin 39 g/ℓ, globulin 27 g/ℓ, bilirubin 9 μmol/ℓ, alkaline phosphatase 89 IU/ℓ, AST 19 IU/ℓ, ALT 16 IU/ℓ and gamma GT 14 IU/ℓ. X-ray of knees and ankles showed minor narrowing of the joint spaces with some calcification in the cartilages of the right knee joint.

Questions

1. What is the diagnosis?
2. State three confirmatory tests.
3. What is the treatment for this condition?

Case 28

A 23-year-old man developed right hypochondrial pain, nausea, jaundice and dark urine. On examination his liver was just palpable. Liver function tests, done by his general practitioner showed a bilirubin of 100 μmol/ℓ, alkaline phosphatase of 250 IU/ℓ and ALT of 800 IU/ℓ. A diagnosis of infective hepatitis was made. Over the next 2 months he improved but complained of mild nausea and persistent jaundice. Repeat liver function tests showed a bilirubin of 75 μmol/ℓ, alkaline phosphatase 175 IU/ℓ, and ALT 82 IU/ℓ. Two months later the jaundice was slightly less, but intermittent nausea persisted. Bilirubin was 50 μmol/ℓ, alkaline phosphatase 100 IU/ℓ, and ALT and gamma GT normal. When seen in the outpatient clinic 6 months after his original illness, the only other symptom elicited was fatigue.

There was no significant past history, the patient was on no drugs and did not drink alcohol. He denied a family history of liver disease. On examination he was slightly jaundiced, but had no lymphadenopathy, spider naevi, or hepatosplenomegaly. Liver function tests were unchanged, the total protein was 76 g/ℓ, albumin 40 g/ℓ, and prothrombin time normal. Hepatitis B surface antigen and auto antibodies were negative.

Questions

1. What is the most likely diagnosis?
2. Which three investigations would be helpful in confirming this?
3. How should he be managed?

Case 29

A 53-year-old tax inspector was referred for investigation of persistent watery diarrhoea. He had suffered from occasional attacks of loose stools since childhood but following a partial gastrectomy for benign gastric ulcer 4 years earlier he had developed more persistent diarrhoea. His symptoms occurred during the mornings and consisted of 3 to 4 moderate sized watery stools associated with abdominal distension and flatulence. He had no other symptoms and denied seeing blood or mucus in the stools. Examination was normal apart from a mid-line abdominal scar and marked perianal excoriation. His full blood count, ESR, serum electrolytes and liver function tests were normal. A 24 hour stool collection weighed 500 g and analysis revealed a pH of 5.7, osmolality of 430 mosmol/kg, sodium of 86 mmol/ℓ and potassium of 65 mmol/ℓ. The faecal fat content of a 3 day collection was 23 mmol/day (on a 100 g fat diet) and stool weight decreased to a mean of 50 g/day during a 3 day fast. Jejunal biopsy was normal on microscopy and no laxatives were detectable in random urine and faecal samples.

Questions

1. What do the results of the stool analyses indicate?
2. What is the most likely diagnosis?
3. List three investigations that may help confirm the diagnosis.
4. What is the relevance of gastric surgery to his symptoms?

Case 30

A 26-year-old policeman was admitted with a 4 week history of watery diarrhoea, up to 10 stools a day. This had begun whilst on holiday in Spain, and was not associated with the passage of blood or mucus. He had lost 13 Kg in weight and on admission was vomiting, lethargic and weak.

Four months prior to admission he had attended another hospital with a swelling involving the vertex of the skull. Excision and histological examination had revealed it to be a malignant deposit but an extensive search for a primary tumour was negative. No definitive histological diagnosis was made.

Serum electrolyte estimation revealed Na^+ 124 mmol/ℓ, K^+ 1.7 mmol/ℓ and Urea 15.4 mmol/ℓ. A 24 hour stool collection yielded 2 litres of watery stool and stool electrolytes were Na^+ 177 mmol/ℓ, K^+ 29 mmol/ℓ and osmolality 275 mosmol/kg. Serum calcium was 3.5 mmol/ℓ.

Questions

1. What is the relevance of the stool electrolyte results?
2. What three tests should be performed in order to establish a diagnosis?
3. How should the patient be managed?

Case 31

A 62-year-old retired school teacher had a 6 month history of inter-mittent, colicky, lower abdominal pain associated with distension and vomiting. She had lost 10 kg in weight and complained of frequent rectal bleeding. For the previous 3 months she had felt progressively lethargic and weak, and had rarely left her home. There was no history of aphthous ulcers, eye, skin or joint symptoms and her past medical history included appendicectomy, migraine and uterine carcinoma, treated by surgery and radiotherapy 15 years previously. She had smoked more than 20 cigarettes a day for the past 30 years but denied ingestion of alcohol. Drug therapy had consisted of a paracetamol–codeine mixture and metoclopramide.

On examination, she was pale and had right lower abdominal tenderness. Sigmoidoscopy showed widespread diffuse telangiectasia, the surrounding mucosa being pale and atrophic. Investigations revealed a haemoglobin of 9.6 g/dl; MCV 111 fl; white count 8.6 × $10^9/\ell$; ESR 31 mm/hour, albumin 31 g/ℓ, calcium 2.0 mmol/ℓ and faecal fat of 36 mmol/day. A barium enema showed a smooth stricture in the caecum but no other abnormality.

Questions

1. Name the two most likely diagnoses?
2. Name two investigations that would help establish the diagnosis?

Case 32

A 53-year-old man was admitted with haematemesis and melaena. He had not experienced abdominal pain or dyspepsia, and had taken no drugs. He drank 2 to 3 pints of beer per week and 4 years previously had undergone a cholecystectomy, with removal of calculi from the common bile duct. During this operation the bile duct was accidentally transected and post-operatively he developed septicaemia and ascites.

On examination he was pale, but there was no jaundice or stigmata of chronic liver disease. His liver was not palpable but the spleen was detected 4 cm below the costal margin. No ascites or hepatic encephalopathy were present. Haemoglobin was 9.6 g/dl, and platelets 103 × $10^9/\ell$. The remainder of the full blood count, electrolytes and liver function tests were normal. Upper gastrointestinal endoscopy confirmed bleeding from oesophageal varices. Wedged hepatic venous pressure was normal.

Questions

1. What is the significance of the normal wedge hepatic venous pressure?
2. What is the probable cause of the portal hypertension?
3. How could the transient ascites following biliary surgery be explained?
4. What investigation would most likely confirm the cause of the portal hypertension?

Case 33

A 56-year-old housewife with long standing rheumatoid arthritis, was admitted to hospital having vomited a 'cupful' of fresh blood and passed melaena stools. She had suffered from intermittent heartburn and flatulence for some 15 years and had derived benefit from antacid mixtures prescribed by her general practitioner. Seropositive rheumatoid arthritis had been diagnosed 20 years earlier and she complained of pain and stiffness involving several joints, especially the metacarpophalangeal, interphalangeal and wrist joints of both hands. On examination, she appeared pale and sweaty, her radial pulse rate was 110/min and her blood pressure 95/60 mmHg. There were deformities of both hands consistent with chronic rheumatoid arthritis and rheumatoid nodules were present on the extensor surfaces of both elbow joints. Abdominal examination revealed moderate epigastric tenderness but there was no rigidity or guarding. Her liver was normal in size and her spleen palpable 1 cm below the left costal margin. Rectal examination revealed black, tarry stools that were strongly positive on Hemoccult testing. Urgent investigations showed a haemoglobin of 8.5 g/dl, MCV of 71 fl, MCHC of 21 g/dl, ESR of 63 mm/hour and normal electrolytes. Urinalysis revealed protein +++ but no other abnormality and routine X-rays of the chest and abdomen were normal.

Questions

1. What two further items of information should be elicited from the history to help diagnose the cause of the bleeding?
2. List three possible causes of splenomegaly in this patient.
3. What would be the two main aims of management during the initial 24 hour period?

Case 34

A 62-year-old factory worker attended his general practitioner because of lethargy and weakness. For 6 months he had noticed gradual deterioration in exercise tolerance because of increasing dyspnoea. Despite a fair appetite, he felt weak and had lost 6 kg over the preceding 2 months. He had no gastrointestinal symptoms apart from postprandial fullness, which had been present for many years. Past medical history included a partial gastrectomy 20 years previously for a benign gastric ulcer and a chronic cough with small amounts of mucoid sputum. His only medication was oral salbutamol (4 mg t.d.s). He smoked 20 cigarettes per day and drank 4 pints of beer a week.

On examination he was pale and thin with slight ankle oedema. The chest was over inflated with scattered inspiratory rhonchi and the abdomen was normal apart from an old surgical scar. Rectal examination revealed only normal coloured stool. Haemoglobin was 7.6 g/dl, MCV 96 fl and MCHC 20 g/dl. Urea and electrolytes, liver function tests and a chest X-ray were normal.

Questions

1. What three mechanisms may be responsible for his anaemia?
2. What four initial investigations are indicated?

Case 35

A 20-year-old electrical engineer had a 6 week history of peri-umbilical abdominal pain, vomiting and diarrhoea. The pain was exacerbated by stress and physical activity and could last several hours at a time. There was no consistent relationship with food but fluids tended to exacerbate the pain. In addition he complained of anorexia, lethargy and weight loss of 5 kg. Two months previously he had returned from a holiday in Greece. His maternal grand-mother had 'colitis' and the patient had recently become engaged to a girl who had a peptic ulcer. He smoked 15 cigarettes a day and recently stopped drinking alcohol. On examination he was slim, pale, febrile (38.8°C) and had tenderness around a vague, central abdominal mass. Rectal examination showed pale fatty stools. The haemoglobin was 10.1 g/ℓ; MCV 82 fl; white count $8.4 \times 10^9/\ell$; ESR 33 mm/hour; albumin 26 g/ℓ; liver function tests normal and faecal fat 44 mmol/day. Sigmoidoscopy with biopsy and chest X-ray were normal. Barium meal and follow-through examination showed wide-spread distortion and fissuring of jejunal mucosa with some dilata-tion of the bowel. The ileum looked normal and barium enema revealed no abnormality.

Questions

1. What two diagnoses should be considered?
2. Name two helpful investigations.

Case 36

A 46-year-old spinster fell downstairs fracturing three ribs. Three weeks later she developed nausea, anorexia, right hypochondrial pain, jaundice, dark urine and pale stools, but no pruritis or rigors. There was no history of fat intolerance or jaundice prior to this episode. She denied taking drugs and only drank alcohol occasionally.

On examination she was obese, had a persistent pyrexia of 38°C and a tachycardia of around 100/min. There was marked jaundice, tenderness in the right hypochondrium, and a positive Murphy's sign. Her gall bladder was not palpable but there was 6 cm hepatomegaly. She had no splenomegaly or ascites. Investigation revealed a bilirubin of 370 μmol/ℓ, alkaline phosphatase 322 IU/ℓ, ALT 50 IU/ℓ, AST 79 IU/ℓ, gamma GT 422 IU/ℓ, total protein 60 g/ℓ and albumin of 29 g/ℓ. Her white cell count was 15.6 × 10^9/ℓ, haemoglobin 10.1 g/dl, MCV 100 fl, and platelets of 90 × 10^9/ℓ. Prothrombin time was prolonged by 7 seconds. An ultrasound scan identified an enlarged but otherwise normal liver, a gallstone in the gallbladder, and a normal biliary tree and pancreas.

Questions

1. What is the most likely diagnosis?
2. What is the most helpful investigation to confirm the diagnosis?
3. Which single investigation correlates best with the prognosis of this condition?

Case 37

A 59-year-old Indian housewife was admitted for investigation of malaise, weight loss of 10 kg and night sweats of 6 months duration. She was unable to speak English and most of the history was obtained from her husband. In addition there was a vague history of recurrent epigastric discomfort and flatulence but she had no other symptoms or past medical history of relevance. The patient had been resident in the UK for 15 years. On examination she was moderately obese, her temperature was 38.5°C and there were small lymph nodes palpable in both axillae. She had a tachycardia of 110/min and abdominal examination revealed moderate obesity and tenderness in the epigastrium and peri-umbilical regions. During the next few days she had an intermittent fever accompanied by rigors and profuse sweating. Haemoglobin was 9.4 g/dl and the blood film revealed normochromic, normocytic red cells and no evidence of malaria. The white cell count ranged from 12.3 to $15.0 \times 10^9/\ell$ with 93% neutrophils and the ESR was 78 mm/hour. Conjugated bilirubin was 96 μmol/ℓ, alkaline phosphatase 350 IU/ℓ and gamma GT 264 IU/ℓ. Chest X-ray and plain abdominal films were normal, urine negative on microscopy and culture (including for acid fast bacilli) and a mantoux test positive (1 in 1000). Bone marrow showed changes of 'chronic disease' only and one of four blood cultures grew gram negative bacilli.

Questions

1. What are the two most likely diagnoses?
2. List three investigations that would be most useful in arriving at the diagnosis.
3. How would you treat these two disorders?

Case 38

A 69-year-old retired boilerman was admitted for investigation. Over the previous year he had lost 12 kg in weight and his ankles had become increasingly swollen. Apart from occasional nausea he had no other symptoms and his bowels were open twice a day with normal looking stools. He was taking no regular medication, was a non-smoker and rarely drank alcohol. There was no relevant family history.

On examination he was thin with generalized muscle wasting, but no other neurological signs. He had marked ankle oedema and a number of small bruises on both legs. A right sided hydrocoele was noted and rectal examination revealed an enlarged prostate.

Haemoglobin, differential white cell count and platelets were normal. Serum calcium was 2.1 mmol/ℓ and alkaline phosphatase 178 IU/ℓ. Bilirubin, liver enzymes and serum electrolytes were normal. Serum albumin was 26 g/ℓ and total protein 53 g/ℓ. Pro-thrombin time was 16 seconds (control 14 seconds) and serum folate was greater than 20 μg/ℓ. Three day faecal fat estimation yielded a fat output of 24 mmol/day. Jejunal biopsy showed a mild inflamma-tory cell infiltrate only. Pancreatic scan was normal and the urine was negative for protein. A plain X-ray of the abdomen showed multiple fluid levels just above the umbilicus.

Questions

1. What diagnosis is suggested by the radiological findings and what investigation would confirm this?
2. What is the significance of the serum folate result and give two tests which would confirm this?

Case 39

A 16-year-old schoolboy presented with a 6 month history of lethargy, nausea and diarrhoea. His bowels were opened 3 times during the day and twice at night, the stools being mushy, pale and offensive. He also had episodes of colicky abdominal pain, 1 – 2 hours after eating, relieved by rest and Buscopan. Recently he had started to fall behind in his schoolwork and had not been fit enough to play in the school football team. Two years previously he had a perianal abscess which had discharged spontaneously but there was no other significant past history. There was a family history of psoriasis and a maternal aunt had been diagnosed as having 'colitis'. On examination he was 169 cm tall, weighed 51.9 kg, and had normal secondary sexual development. Abdominal examination revealed some tenderness to the right of the midline and an anal skin tag.

Investigations showed a haemoglobin of 10.3 g/ℓ, MCV 67 fl, ESR 25 mm/hour, serum folate 0.2 μg/ℓ, red cell folate 84 μg/ℓ, serum B$_{12}$ 280 ng/ℓ, serum iron 5 μmol/ℓ and TIBC 60 μmol/ℓ. Barium follow-through examination showed coarse duodenal and jejunal folds and a normal ileum. Jejunal biopsy demonstrated slight shortening of the villi, lengthening of the crypts and marked neutrophil and eosinophil infiltration of the lamina propria. An endoscopy to the 2nd part of the duodenum was normal.

Questions

1. What is the most likely diagnosis?
2. Name two most helpful investigations.
3. What are the two principle aims of management of this case?

Case 40

A 35-year-old Estate Agent presented with a 2 year history of diarrhoea passing three or four pale, loose motions per day, weight loss of 2 stone, recurrent mouth ulceration, lethargy, and tiredness. In addition he had a long history of chronic sinusitis, and a 10 year history of winter bronchitis. There was no history of abdominal pain. Three years previously he had been on holiday to France and Spain. He drank one whisky per day, did not smoke, and had no relevant family history. Loperamide, as required for the diarrhoea, was the only medication taken.

On examination he was thin and pale, had no lymphadenopathy and no abnormal abdominal findings. Haemoglobin was 8.6 g/dl, MCV 101 fl, serum vitamin B$_{12}$ 96 ng/ℓ, serum folate 4.0 μg/ℓ, and gastric parietal cell and intrinsic factor antibodies were negative. Total protein was 50 g/ℓ, albumin 30 g/ℓ, iron 6 μmol/ℓ, TIBC 21 μmol/ℓ, 5 hour urinary xylose recovery 20%, and faecal fat 44 mmol/day. Urea, electrolytes, liver function tests, prothrombin time and corrected calcium were normal. Microscopy and culture of faeces detected no pathogens. A barium meal and follow-through showed a normal stomach, but appearances of 'nodular lymphoid hyperplasia' in the jejunum.

Questions

1. What is the most likely diagnosis?
2. What three investigations would be helpful to confirm this?
3. What are two possible mechanisms for the anaemia?

Case 41

A 78-year-old male diabetic was admitted urgently to hospital because of fever, malaise and right hypochondrial pain. He had been well until 24 hours prior to admission when he developed sudden onset of abdominal pain radiating into his back. This was severe and associated with nausea and vomiting. A few hours after the onset of these symptoms he felt feverish and developed rigors. He had been an insulin-requiring diabetic for 23 years. On examination, he appeared ill and flushed with a temperature of 39.5°C. His pulse rate was 120/min, blood pressure 90/60 mmHg and he was dehydrated. Abdominal examination revealed marked tenderness in the right hypochondrium and epigastrium with guarding, and on deep palpation there was a vague mass in the right upper quadrant. He was slightly tender in the right loin but the remainder of the examination was unremarkable. Haemoglobin was 11.2 g/dl, WBC 28.5 $\times$ $10^9/\ell$ with 90% neutrophils, ESR 69 mm/hour, urea 17.5 mmol/ℓ, HCO_3^- 15 mmol/ℓ and blood glucose 28.0 mmol/ℓ. Bilirubin was 34 μmol/ℓ, AST 55 IU/ℓ and alkaline phosphatase 205 IU/ℓ. His urine contained protein, glucose, ketones and bilirubin. Urine microscopy revealed 50 WBC per high power field but no bacteria, and his chest X-ray and ECG were normal. Erect abdominal film was normal although curious gas shadows were noted in the vicinity of the gall bladder. An ultrasound scan showed normal liver but the gall bladder was not visualized.

Questions

1. What two related diagnoses may be made in the above patient?
2. What further investigations should be performed to confirm the cause of his abdominal symptoms?
3. List three priorities in treating this patient during the initial 24 hour period.

Case 42

A 28-year-old British physician was taken ill whilst attending a medical conference in Mexico. After 4 days at the conference he developed diarrhoea, passing 12 watery stools a day, each one preceded by colicky lower abdominal pain. He became feverish and extremely lethargic. Within 12 hours he was unable to get out of bed and began vomiting bile stained fluid. Four years prior to this trip he had complained of diarrhoea with blood and mucus, and ulcerative colitis had been diagnosed on sigmoidoscopy and barium enema. Since that time he had been taking Salazopyrine 1 g b.d. orally and had been free of bowel symptoms.

On admission to the local hospital he was pyrexial (38°C) and dehydrated. Abdominal examination was normal and the rectum was empty. Haemoglobin was 17 g/dl and blood film normal. Other blood tests revealed a serum Na^+ of 149 mmol/ℓ, serum K^+ of 3.0 mmol/ℓ and blood urea of 13 mmol/ℓ. Sigmoidoscopy showed a granular mucosa and watery stool but no blood or mucus.

Questions

1. What is the most likely cause of his diarrhoea?
2. What three measures could have prevented it?
3. What three therapeutic measures should be taken?

Case 43

A 60-year-old retired furnaceman was referred to the out-patient clinic with an 18 month history of faecal incontinence, usually at night. His bowels were opened once or twice a day, and the stools were watery with streaks of fresh blood. He admitted to some perianal discomfort but there was no abdominal pain, anorexia or weight loss. In the past he had suffered a right sided stroke from which he had fully recovered. Drug therapy consisted of atenolol for hypertension. His wife had been dead for 2 years and he lived with his unmarried, 35-year-old son. On examination he was noted to be unkempt but otherwise well. Blood pressure was 180/100 mmHg.

Cardiac, respiratory and abdominal examinations were unremarkable. Examination of his perineum revealed large fleshy skin tags with three anal sinuses discharging faeces. The perianal skin on the right side was boggy and excoriated and this appearance extended to the anterior superior iliac spine. Rectal examination revealed an irregular anal margin with abnormal mucosa but no stenosis. Proctoscopy revealed a lateral anal fissure and barium enema examination showed irregular rectal mucosa to 3 cm and then normal looking bowel to caecum.

Questions

1. What are the three most likely diagnoses?
2. Name the two most helpful investigations.
3. What is the significance of the lateral fissure?

Case 44

A 32-year-old nurse developed malaise, fatigue, anorexia, nausea, and intermittent fever of 38°C. Two days later she complained of right hypochondrial pain, jaundice, pale motions, dark urine, and pruritis. A week previously she had been diagnosed as having campylobacter enteritis and given a course of erythromycin with good effect. She had received this antibiotic previously, for an episode of bronchitis, without any adverse reactions. There was no other past history, she denied fat intolerance, and took no other medication.

On examination, pyrexia and jaundice were confirmed, but there were no stigmata of chronic liver disease and no lymphadenopathy. She was tender in the right upper quadrant, but the liver and gall bladder were not palpable. Bilirubin was 85 μmol/ℓ, alkaline phosphatase 176 IU/ℓ, ALT 123 IU/ℓ, gamma GT 197 IU/ℓ and albumin 38 g/ℓ. The total white cell count was 12.5 $\times$ 10^9/ℓ with atypical lymphocytes on the blood film. Plain abdominal X-ray was normal.

Questions

1. List three possible diagnoses.
2. What three investigations are indicated?

Case 45

A 12-year-old schoolboy was referred because of weakness, tiredness, weight loss of 4 kg and generalized oedema. He admitted to slight intermittent ankle oedema for about 1 year and in recent months this had spread to involve the whole of his legs, face and hands. His appetite remained fair and a detailed diet history confirmed adequate calorie and protein intake. On questioning he complained of intermittent diarrhoea and the stools were often pale in appearance and difficult to flush away. Six weeks prior to referral his general practitioner had prescribed a strict gluten free diet, without obvious improvement. Examination confirmed the presence of generalized, asymetrical oedema with involvement of both lower limbs. His height and weight were just above the third percentile, abdominal examination was normal and rectal examination revealed the presence of soft, pale stools with a foul odour. Investigations showed a haemoglobin of 12.8 g/dl, WBC of $6.3 \times 10^9/\ell$ (differential count: 85% neutrophils, 7% lymphocytes, 7% monocytes and 1% eosinophils). Serum urea, electrolytes and creatinine were normal, albumin 23 g/ℓ, total protein 46 g/ℓ, alkaline phosphatase 163 IU/ℓ, ALT 25 IU/ℓ and gamma GT 35 IU/ℓ. Immunoglobulin estimation showed an IgG of 3.9 g/ℓ, IgM of 0.30 g/ℓ and IgA of 0.5 g/ℓ. Urinalysis showed a trace of protein, and urine microscopy was normal.

Questions

1. What is the most likely explanation for his biochemical abnormalities and how may this be confirmed?
2. What is the pathological diagnosis and the best method for confirming this?
3. How would you treat the patient?

Case 46

A 37-year-old engineer was transferred from the orthopaedic unit with acute upper gastrointestinal bleeding. He had been admitted for revision surgery of an infected, low friction arthroplasty of the right hip. Previously an osteotomy had been performed on the left hip and he had a splenectomy at the age of 11 years. He had been taking soluble aspirin and cephradine regularly for several months prior to admission. There was no history of jaundice and he drank little alcohol. An older sister had a splenectomy at the age of 7 years because of a bleeding tendency.

On examination he was pale but not shocked, the liver was enlarged 3 fingerbreadths below the costal margin and there was a discharging sinus in the right groin. X-rays of both hips revealed flattening of the femoral head on the left and a loosened hip prosthesis on the right with evidence of infection. Emergency endoscopy revealed bleeding lower oesophageal varices. Haemoglobin was 9.6 g/dl, MCV 80 fl and MCHC 33 g/dl. Blood urea was 8.3 mmol/ℓ and electrolytes were normal. Acid phosphatase was 14.9 IU/ℓ, serum albumin 30 g/ℓ, AST 67 IU/ℓ and gamma GT 106 IU/ℓ.

Questions

1. What is the likely cause of his portal hypertension?
2. What is the relevance of the family history?
3. Give three non-surgical methods of arresting the acute bleeding.

Case 47

An 18-year-old barmaid was admitted to hospital with a 12 hour history of progressive, central abdominal pain accompanied by vomiting and abdominal distension. She had just returned from Scotland where she had been on a week's holiday with her boyfriend. Apart from being diagnosed as having asthma 6 months previously (poorly controlled on a salbutamol inhaler) she had no other relevant history and denied abdominal symptoms prior to this episode. There was a family history of eczema and hay fever and she was not on the contraceptive pill. On examination she was in pain and clinically shocked, with a pulse of 120/min and blood pressure of 85/50 mmHg. There was marked abdominal tenderness, muscle guarding and rigidity, and absent bowel sounds. Investigations showed a haemoglobin of 10.4 g/dl; white blood count of 12.6 × 10^9/ℓ (70% neutrophils, 20% lymphocytes, 3% monocytes, 7% eosinophils) and

ESR of 88 mm/hour. Blood film showed normochromic and normocytic red cells. Sodium was 128 mmol/ℓ, potassium 3.0 mmol/ℓ and urea 10 mmol/ℓ. Plain abdominal X-ray showed dilated loops of small bowel with numerous fluid levels. Chest X-ray was normal, FEV_1 was 2.4 ℓ and peak flow rate 170 ℓ/min. Routine testing of her urine revealed proteinuria. After initial resuscitation with intravenous fluids, a laparotomy was performed which demonstrated extensive small bowel infarction. The infarcted bowel was resected leaving her with about 40 cm of duodenum which was anastomosed to the ascending colon. Post-operatively she suffered recurrent attacks of supraventricular arrhythmias.

Questions

1. What is the diagnosis?
2. What treatment would you advocate for this disease?
3. What is the likely complication of her surgery and how should this be managed?

Case 48

A 31-year-old bank clerk developed an upper respiratory tract infection, for which she was prescribed ampicillin. Four days later she developed semi-solid motions containing mucus, four times per day. One week later her bowel frequency increased to 12 times per day and on most occasions the stool contained fresh red blood. She also experienced left iliac fossa pain relieved by defaecation. Other symptoms included malaise, tiredness and aching of her knees, wrists and fingers. Although she had not lost weight, she complained of anorexia and nausea. Over the previous 4 years the patient had experienced several acute, self-limiting attacks of blood-stained diarrhoea.

On examination she was dehydrated, pale, pyrexial (38°C), had a pulse of 104/min and blood pressure of 115/70 mmHg. Her abdomen was tender in the left iliac fossa but there was no palpable mass and bowel sounds were normal. On digital examination, the anal canal was narrow and tender and blood stained, semi-solid faeces were present in the rectum. Investigations showed a haemoglobin of 11.3

g/dl, white cell count·15 × $10^9/\ell$, ESR 48 mm/hour, urea 7.6 mmol/ℓ, normal electrolytes, total protein 60 g/ℓ and albumin 28 g/ℓ. Plain abdominal X-ray was normal and microbiological studies on her stools negative. Despite intensive medical therapy she continued to feel unwell, with blood stained diarrhoea 12 – 14 times per day, a pyrexia and persistent tachycardia. Her haemoglobin fell to 9.1 g/dl and albumin to 24 g/ℓ.

Questions

1. List four possible diagnoses and state which is most likely.
2. What three further investigations would be helpful in confirming the diagnosis in this patient?
3. State three clinical features, in this patient, that indicate the need for surgical intervention.

Case 49

A 50-year-old housewife was referred to the medical out-patient clinic because of persistent watery diarrhoea and faecal incontinence which had been present for 8 years. Her bowels were opened six times per day and she frequently experienced incontinence of liquid faeces. The stools were occasionally pale, offensive and difficult to flush away. She complained of post-prandial fullness and nausea, occasionally accompanied by sweating and palpitations. Further enquiry revealed occasional attacks of facial flushing and sweating related to eating. She had no contact with patients suffering from diarrhoea but had been on holiday in Turkey 6 years previously. In the past she had 2 children delivered by forceps, had a cholecystectomy at the age of 35 years and a vagotomy and pyloroplasty 3 years later. Examination showed a thin, pale woman with a fine tremor of both hands and rather sweaty palms. There were no stigmata of gastrointestinal disease and abdominal examination was normal. Rectal examination revealed a lax anal sphincter and the presence of watery stools. Investigations showed a normal full blood count, ESR and liver function tests. Serum potassium was 2.9 mmol/ℓ, sodium 134 mmol/ℓ and urea 3.6 mmol/ℓ. Stool weight was 450 g/day and faecal fat content 24 mmol/day. Stools were consistently negative for pathogens, occult blood and laxatives.

Questions

1. What are the two major factors responsible for the diarrhoea and mild steatorrhoea?
2. What is the cause of her flushing, sweating and palpitations?
3. What three further investigations would help define the cause of this patient's diarrhoea?

Case 50

A 49-year-old driver was admitted with jaundice. He had a 9 month history of episodic watery diarrhoea, without blood or mucus and occasional attacks of nocturnal diarrhoea. During this period he often felt flushed, sweaty, and dyspnoeic and had lost a few pounds in weight. For 4 months he had suffered from intermittent epigastric and right upper quadrant pain, helped a little by cimetidine. One week before admission he had become markedly jaundiced with severe itching, discoloured urine and stools.

On examination he was jaundiced, had scratch marks on the skin and telangiectasia on the face. There was a systolic murmur heard loudest in the pulmonary area and he was tender on deep palpation in the right upper quadrant of the abdomen. Rectal examination revealed only pale stools. Serum bilirubin was 153 μmol/ℓ and alkaline phosphatase 1325 IU/ℓ. Total protein was 73 g/ℓ, albumin 43 g/ℓ and gamma GT 919 IU/ℓ. Hepatitis BsAg was negative and prothrombin time 14 seconds (control 13 seconds). Ultrasound scan of the liver showed dilated intrahepatic ducts and percutaneous transhepatic cholangiography revealed a short stricture at the porta hepatis with contrast passing slowly into a normal common bile duct.

Questions

1. What is the most likely diagnosis?
2. What two tests may confirm the diagnosis?
3. What four treatment options are available?

Case 51

A 21-year-old male nurse presented with a 2 month history of diarrhoea, up to 8 times a day, accompanied by blood and mucus. He developed anorexia and lost about 2.5 kg in weight. For the previous fortnight he had felt increasingly lethargic but denied any abdominal pain. Two weeks before his symptoms started the patient had returned from a holiday in Yugoslavia but while there he had been well and had no contact with any diarrhoeal illness. There was a past history of asthma treated with slow release theophylline and beclomethasone inhaler. Both his father and grandfather had suffered from duodenal ulcer. He was unmarried, shared a flat with a fellow nurse, and had worked on a respiratory ward for nearly 3 years. On examination he was slim and pale. His descending colon was palpable but not tender. Rectal examination revealed blood on the glove and sigmoidoscopy showed a loss of vascular pattern with erythema, contact bleeding and a patchy exudate involving the distal 5 cm and normal mucosa above this. His haemoglobin was 9.9 g/dl, MCV 71 fl, WBC $10.0 \times 10^9/\ell$, and ESR 45 mm/hour. Urea, serum electrolytes and liver function tests were normal. Plain abdominal X-ray showed faecal residues in the transverse and descending colon.

Questions

1. What is the diagnosis?
2. Name three helpful investigations.
3. What 2 drugs would you use to treat this disorder?

Case 52

A 67-year-old lady was first noticed to be jaundiced by her daughter. Within 1 week the jaundice became marked and was associated with generalized pruritis, dark urine and pale motions. She denied fever or rigors. Over the past few weeks her appetite had decreased and she thought she had lost weight. Five years previously she had undergone a cholecystectomy with removal of gallstones from the common bile duct.

On examination she was apyrexial and markedly jaundiced. There were no spider naevi and no lymphadenopathy. Widespread scratch marks were present and she had 4 cm hepatomegaly. The abdomen was non-tender and there was no evidence of a mass or palpable gall bladder.

Bilirubin was 345 μmol/ℓ, alkaline phosphatase 430 IU/ℓ, gamma GT 150 IU/ℓ, ALT 75 IU/ℓ and albumin 32 g/ℓ. The prothrombin time, which was initially 3 seconds prolonged, was corrected by vitamin K injections. Plain abdominal X-ray was normal. Ultrasound scan showed normal liver parenchyma and dilated intrahepatic ducts, but failed to outline the common bile duct.

Questions

1. List four possible diagnoses.
2. Of these diagnoses, which would be most compatible with the ultrasound result?
3. What three investigations could be used to confirm the diagnosis?
4. What two treatment options are available for this?

Case 53

A 73-year-old retired coalminer attended his general practitioner because of weakness, malaise, anorexia and weight loss of 6 kg. There was a long standing history of chronic obstructive airways disease and his current symptoms developed over a period of 3 months. He had a daily cough productive of mucoid sputum and was dyspnoeic on moderate exertion. Physical examination revealed a thin man with evidence of 'coal tattooing' and pallor. There was no peripheral lymphadenopathy and cardiorespiratory examination showed widespread expiratory rhonchi but no other abnormality. Abdominal inspection revealed divarication of the recti and peri-umbilical visible peristalsis. His sigmoid colon was palpable and a vague mass was felt in the right iliac fossa. Haemoglobin was 8.2 g/dl with an MCV of 64 fl and MCHC of 21 g/dl; ESR 78 mm/hour, total protein 65 g/ℓ, albumin 33 g/ℓ, alkaline phosphatase 195 IU/ℓ, and electrolytes were normal. Chest X-ray showed emphysematous changes in the lower lobes and calcified hilar lymph nodes 'consistent with old tuberculosis'. One of three stool samples was positive for occult blood. Barium meal was normal and barium enema showed extensive sigmoid diverticula with 'faecal material in the caecal pole'. The patient was subsequently referred to a local hospital for a further opinion.

Questions

1. What is the most likely diagnosis?
2. How would you confirm the presence of this disease?
3. Name two pathological entities that predispose to the development of this condition.
4. In the above patient, what two factors may influence his further management?

Case 54

A 60-year-old man was admitted as an emergency complaining of abdominal pain. He had attended his general practitioner on several occasions during the previous 6 months complaining of colicky lower abdominal pain and diarrhoea, without rectal bleeding. As a result he had been advised to take a high fibre diet. Six hours prior to admission he developed similar abdominal pain which gradually became worse and was associated with marked tenesmus. He had previously been well and was employed in a steel foundry, until forced to retire early because of chronic bronchitis and emphysema. A right inguinal hernia was repaired 10 years previously and his appendix was removed at the age of 22 years. His only regular medication was a long acting, oral bronchodilator.

On examination he was apyrexial, and was breathing through pursed lips. His chest was overexpanded but otherwise normal. The abdomen was distended and tympanitic, and there was slight tenderness in the left iliac fossa but no rebound tenderness. Bowel sounds were present and active, and hernial orifices clear. Rectal examination was normal and sigmoidoscopy showed several bluish, sessile polyps in the rectum. Full blood count and serum electrolytes were normal. Straight X-ray of the abdomen showed gas in a dilated colon with a few fluid levels. In addition there were multiple gas bubbles present in the left iliac fossa.

Questions

1. What is the clinical diagnosis and the most likely cause?
2. What are the two most commonly associated disorders?
3. What two medical treatments are available?

Case 55

A 58-year-old drayman was admitted for investigation of weight loss. He had lost 19 kg in 18 months and in addition complained of lethargy and weakness. There was no history of anorexia or abdominal pain. His bowels were opened 4 times a day and the stools were pale in colour. He had noticed recent ankle oedema and discomfort in his left foot and both wrists. Six months prior to admission, he and his family had been on holiday to Spain but his family had remained well. There was a past history of rheumatic fever and appendicitis and he intermittently took soluble aspirin. On examination, he was wasted (weight 41 kg), pyrexial (39°C) and had moderately enlarged, non-tender lymph glands in both axillae and groins. There was mild generalized pigmentation, the blood pressure was 105/60 mmHg and an ejection systolic murmur was heard over the left sternal edge. His abdomen was distended but there was no organomegaly or masses. Examination of the musculo-skeletal system showed widespread, asymmetrical, small joint arthropathy and a swollen, tender right first metacarpophalangeal joint.

Investigations showed a haemoglobin of 8.1 g/ℓ, MCV 66 fl and white cell count 8.0 × 10^9/ℓ (differential normal). Blood film showed microcytosis and his ESR was 85 mm/hour. Albumin was 30 g/ℓ, globulin 40 g/ℓ, bilirubin 5 μmol/ℓ, alkaline phosphatase 60 IU/ℓ, AST 15 IU/ℓ, ALT 29 IU/ℓ, and gamma GT 26 IU/ℓ.

Questions

1. What is the most likely diagnosis?
2. Name three most useful investigations.
3. What is the treatment?

Case 56

A 22-year-old university student developed malaise, anorexia, nausea and right upper abdominal discomfort, followed by dark urine, pale stools, and jaundice. He had no pruritis or rigors. After 3 weeks, his symptoms and jaundice resolved, only to recur 1 month later. Six weeks prior to his illness he had been re-united with his girlfriend, who had recently developed jaundice while on holiday in Egypt. He drank 35 pints of beer per week and denied abusing intravenous drugs or having homosexual relationships.

On examination, he was markedly jaundiced had 2 small cervical lymph nodes, but no cutaneous stigmata of liver disease. His liver was enlarged by 6 cm and spleen by 4 cm. There was no evidence of ascites or hepatic encephalopathy. Haemoglobin was 14.5 g/dl, white cell count $4.6 \times 10^9/\ell$, with a relative lymphocytosis including atypical forms. Bilirubin was 323 μmol/ℓ, alkaline phosphatase 250 IU/ℓ, ALT 1380 IU/ℓ, globulin 50 g/ℓ, albumin 43 g/ℓ, and prothrombin time was 11 seconds prolonged.

Questions

1. What is the most likely diagnosis?
2. What three blood tests may help to establish the precise cause of his hepatic dysfunction?

Case 57

A 77-year-old Indian was admitted urgently to hospital complaining of severe left side abdominal pain. He was unable to speak English and most of the history was obtained through his daughter. The pain had started suddenly while straining at stool, 4 hours prior to admission. Discomfort was maximal over the left lower quadrant and periumbilical region and he described the pain as continuous. His bowels were opened on alternate days and normal stool had been passed approximately 14 hours before admission. No faecal material or flatus had been passed since the onset of the pain. For 8 months prior to admission he had experienced several attacks of acute left iliac fossa pain and abdominal distension lasting 3 – 4 hours. Recovery had been spontaneous and was followed by the passage of liquid stools, mucus and flatus. On examination he was sweaty, and in obvious pain. There was no evidence of anaemia or lymphadenopathy, his pulse rate was 110/min and blood pressure 160/105 mmHg. Cardiorespiratory systems were normal and abdominal inspection revealed a left herniorraphy scar, marked abdominal distension with particular involvement of the left lower quadrant and periumbilical regions. Percussion was tympanitic over these areas and bowel sounds hyperactive. Digital examination revealed an empty rectum. A loud bruit was present over the epigastrium and he had a weak left sided femoral pulse with absent pulses in the left leg. Abdominal X-rays showed a grossly dilated colon containing faecal material and air.

Questions

1. What is the most likely diagnosis?
2. List three differential diagnoses.
3. How is the diagnosis usually confirmed?
4. How would you treat the above patient?

Case 58

A 55-year-old Jamaican was admitted to hospital with a 3 month history of recurrent attacks of nausea, vomiting, abdominal distension and upper abdominal pain. These symptoms occurred immediately after meals and were partly relieved by vomiting. In between attacks he had diarrhoea, three times a day, which he described as pale, frothy and offensive. He had lost 6 kg in weight over the 3 month period. For 1 year prior to admission he had suffered from heartburn and acid reflux, and for 2 years had stiffness of his fingers, with difficulty performing tasks requiring fine movements.

Physical examination revealed thickening of the fingers, and he was unable to form a proper fist due to limitation of flexion. He was thin, with generalized muscle wasting. The abdomen was distended with slight epigastric tenderness but no rebound tenderness. Bowel sounds were normal. Straight abdominal X-ray showed gaseous distension of small bowel, colon and rectum and a barium follow-through examination revealed gross dilatation of the jejunum and proximal ileum with no evidence of mechanical obstruction. Three day faecal fat estimation showed an output of 35 mmol/day and D-Xylose absorption was substantially reduced. Serum folate was 1 μg/ℓ and B_{12} was normal.

Questions

1. What is the diagnosis?
2. Name two further helpful gastrointestinal investigations.
3. What two therapeutic measures are most likely to improve his diarrhoea?

Case 59

A 70-year-old housewife presented to the out-patient clinic with a 3 year history of progressive dysphagia. This occurred mostly after solid food but occasionally developed after drinking fluid. The temperature of ingested material made no difference to the symptoms. The dysphagia occurred within a few minutes of swallowing (food appearing to stick above the sternal notch) and was relieved by vomiting. Her recent appetite had been poor and she had lost 1.5 kg in weight. There was a past history of a cholecystectomy and appendicectomy and the patient had maturity onset diabetes, angina, hypertension, osteoarthritis and psoriasis. Drug therapy included atenolol, nifedipine, metformin, Neonaclex K, GTN and aspirin.

On examination she was obese (78.5 kg), and hypertensive (200/110 mmHg), with an aortic sclerotic murmur. Abdominal examination was normal. There were signs of osteoarthritis affecting the knees and ankles but the remainder of the examination was normal. Investigations revealed a haemoglobin of 12.1 g/dl, MCV 85 fl, ESR 3 mm/hour and white count 6.0 $\times$ 10^9/ℓ. ECG and Chest X-ray were normal.

Questions

1. List three causes of her dysphagia.
2. Name the two most helpful investigations.
3. What is the treatment of choice of the most likely diagnosis?

Case 60

A 73-year-old woman developed increasing jaundice, pale stools and dark urine without pruritus or rigors. Her appetite remained good, she had not lost weight and denied any abdominal pain or dyspepsia. She was on Dyazide and digoxin for atrial fibrillation. There was no past history of jaundice or hepatitis, she rarely drank alcohol and was a non-smoker.

On examination she was afebrile but markedly jaundiced. She had no cutaneous stigmata of liver disease or lymphadenopathy. The abdomen was not tender, there was a palpable mass in the right upper quadrant and rectal examination suggested steatorrhoea. The remainder of the examination was normal apart from the presence of controlled atrial fibrillation. Her initial investigations showed bilirubinuria, serum bilirubin of 376 μmol/ℓ, alkaline phosphatase 363 IU/ℓ, ALT 133 IU/ℓ, and gamma GT 529 IU/ℓ. Total protein, albumin, and prothrombin time were normal. Plain abdominal X-ray showed no gallstones or pancreatic calcification but there was a soft tissue shadow in the right hypochondrium. Full blood count was normal and faecal occult bloods negative.

Questions

1. What are the three most likely diagnoses?
2. What is the significance of the right hypochondrial mass?
3. In the above case, what would be the next investigation of choice?

2   Discussion of cases

Case 1

Answers

1. Multiple pyogenic liver abscesses.
2. Ultrasound scan with guided aspiration.

Discussion

Although tumour metastases is the commonest cause of hepatic space occupying lesions in the UK and Europe, the associated sigmoid diverticular abscess makes pyogenic abscesses the likely diagnosis in this patient. The clinical features in both diseases may be similar and the prognosis equally poor if diagnosis is delayed. The investigation most likely to confirm the nature of the liver disease is ultrasound guided needle aspiration of a hypoechoic lesion. This was performed on the above patient and yielded 60 ml of pus containing streptococcus milleri. A guided liver biopsy (percutaneous or laparoscopic) may show histological evidence of a pyogenic abscess but bacteriological diagnosis is less frequently obtained and this technique is not the investigation of choice in such a patient.

Pyogenic liver abscess is found in 1% of postmortem examinations and accounts for only 0.03% of hospital admissions. Abscesses are usually multiple and the biliary tree is the most frequent source of primary infection. Other sources of infection include septicaemia, trauma, portal pyelophlebitis and extension from adjacent viscera. A number of organisms have been isolated from these abscesses; streptococcus milleri (most common), anaerobic organisms and *E. coli* being common. As illustrated by the present case, the symptoms and signs are often non-specific and blood cultures negative. Fever only occurs in 25% of cases, leucocytosis in half and abnormalities of the right hemidiaphragm and right lower lobe on chest X-ray in 50%. A low albumin and elevated alkaline phosphatase are common and space occupying lesions in the liver are present on ultrasound, CT and isotope scans.

The treatment of pyogenic liver abscess is controversial. Most would advocate parenteral antibiotics, with or without repeated percutaneous aspiration of the larger cavities, in patients with multiple lesions. The choice of antibiotic depends on the organism involved; *streptococcus milleri* being invariably sensitive to benzyl penicillin and resistant to metronidazole, and the other organisms being sensitive to aminoglycosides and metronidazole. If the abscesses fail to resolve on this therapy, open surgical drainage is advocated and some believe this to be the treatment of choice in solitary pyogenic abscess. The patient was treated with parenteral cefuroxime, because of penicillin allergy, and made a recovery with resolution of the hypoechoic lesions within 6 weeks. Repeated aspiration was not performed and in most cases aspiration need only be performed to obtain bacteriological diagnosis.

The mortality of multiple pyogenic liver abscess varies from 10 to 40%. However, if patients are diagnosed early and appropriate antibiotics prescribed the mortality is less than 10%. Therefore, clinical suspicion of hepatic abscess coupled with appropriate investigations are essential in managing such patients.

Case 2

Answers

1. Antibiotic associated colitis.
2. (a) Stool culture for *Clostridium difficile*.
   (b) Stool cytotoxicity.
   (c) Rectal biopsy.
3. Vancomycin.

Discussion

Several diagnoses must be considered in this patient. Diarrhoea in a previously constipated patient is frequently due to faecal impaction, but the severity of the illness and the empty rectum exclude this diagnosis. Acute ulcerative colitis can occur at any age and can rapidly lead to hypoalbuminaemia, hypokalaemia and dehydration. It would however be most unusual for acute ulcerative colitis to present without blood in the stools. Crohn's colitis is a possibility and can present without rectal bleeding, but the sigmoidoscopic appearances are not typical. A patient presenting with a short history of diarrhoea with exudates on the rectal mucosa following antibiotic therapy strongly suggests antibiotic-associated colitis (AAC or pseudomembranous colitis).

AAC is now known to be due chiefly to proliferation of toxin-producing *Clostridium difficile* in the colon. *Clostridium difficile* can be cultured from the stools in 4% of normal adults but its growth is usually inhibited by normal colonic bacterial flora. Patients given antibiotics which suppress the normal gut flora may develop *Cl. difficile* infection and colonic damage. It is said that AAC is more likely to occur in previously constipated individuals because of longer contact times between toxin and mucosa. Many antibiotics have been incriminated, especially clindamycin and ampicillin. AAC is rare in patients given erythromycin or aminoglycosides.

Patients usually present with diarrhoea without bleeding or perforation. Two-thirds of patients have fever and 75% have a low serum albumin. Abdominal cramps and a leucocytosis are also common features. No single feature or test is diagnostic and only 50% of cases have classical sigmoidoscopic appearances. Typical histology showing focal necrosis is obtained by biopsying the edge of a pseudomembranous plaque, but is seen in only 70% of cases. Cytotoxicity tests on stools reveal toxin in almost 80% and *Clostridium difficile* can be cultured in about 90% of cases. The diagnosis is thus made on cumulative evidence from the clinical features, sigmoidoscopic appearances, stool culture and identification of toxin in the stool. In our patient, a low platelet count precluded a rectal biopsy, but stool cultures and cytotoxicity tests were positive.

In the treatment of AAC, repletion of fluid and electrolytes is important and the most effective drug therapy is oral vancomycin, 500 mg q.d.s., although metronidazole has also been used with good results. Cholestyramine binds toxin in the gut, but is not adequate treatment on its own. *Clostridium difficile* is suppressed by antibiotic therapy but may form spores which are not destroyed by vancomycin. When therapy is discontinued the spores may revert to vegetative forms causing clinical relapse. AAC has a mortality of 27%, particularly in patients over 60 years. Our patient deteriorated rapidly despite treatment, and died 2 days later. She proved to be the first of a series of 12 cases in the same haematology unit. Several similar 'mini' epidemics have been reported previously.

Case 3

Answers

1. (a) Laxative abuse.
   (b) VIP secreting tumour of pancreas.
   (c) Crohn's disease.
2. (a) Laxative screen.
   (b) Plasma VIP.
   (c) Jejunal biopsy.

Discussion

A female with persistent diarrhoea resistant to investigation and treatment and accompanied by hypokalaemia suggests either laxative abuse or a VIP secreting pancreatic lesion. Less likely diagnoses include lactose intolerance, diffuse small bowel Crohn's disease and coeliac disease. Helpful investigations would, therefore, include a laxative screen, rectal biopsy for melanosis coli, plasma hormone profile, and jejunal biopsy to exclude jejunal Crohn's disease, coeliac disease and hypolactasia.

Investigations on this lady showed positive urine tests for senna and phenolphthalein. A locker search revealed the presence of laxatives as well as a large quantity of sodium bicarbonate powder, which may well have contributed to her alkalosis.

The diagnosis of laxative abuse is often missed as it is rarely suspected. Ninety-eight per cent of patients are female and appear prepared to put up with any amount of discomfort and hazardous procedures while being investigated. A past psychiatric history and previous history of constipation are frequent findings. Useful indications of laxative abuse include hypokalaemia and melanosis coli. In gross cases, the latter is apparent at proctoscopy or sigmoidoscopy, but in mild cases a rectal biopsy is required. Abuse of anthracene-type laxatives such as senna, cascara and aloes cause this abnormality and it may be detected as early as 4 months after the onset of consumption and disappears within 12 months of withdrawal. In 30% of cases the barium enema shows the presence of 'cathartic colon' in which the bowel is dilated and hypomotile with loss of haustral pattern. Pseudostrictures caused by spasm, lasting many hours, are often seen involving the right side of the colon or even the terminal ileum.

Once suspected, urine and faeces should be sent for analysis. Phenolphthalein and aloes are easily detected by acidification of urine and a simple qualititative urine test for senna is available. Osmotic purgatives contain magnesium, which can be detected in excess quantities in stool specimens (calcium chloride precipitation test). Some patients with laxative abuse also take diuretics and in these a high urine output and urinary sodium may be a clue. The long term prognosis of laxative abuse is guarded as many patients either reject the diagnosis or refuse psychotherapy. Continued psychiatric support and correction of any fluid and electrolyte imbalances are the mainstay of treatment.

Case 4

Answers

1. (a) Peutz–Jegher Syndrome is most likely
   (b) Crohn's disease
2. Accurate family history.
3. (a) Intussusception.
   (b) Gastrointestinal bleeding.
   (c) Increase in gastrointestinal adenocarcinoma.

Discussion

The colicky central abdominal pain suggests small bowel obstruction. This, together with the right iliac fossa mass, is suggestive of small bowel Crohn's disease. The iron deficiency anaemia makes an appendix abscess an unlikely cause, while the mass tends to exclude duodenal ulcer and acute pancreatitis. The presence of mucocutaneous pigmentation makes Peutz–Jegher Syndrome the most likely diagnosis. This is usually inherited as an autosomal dominant condition and an accurate family history should be obtained. Often no other members of the family appear to be affected. In addition to pigmentation, this disorder is associated with hamartomatous polyps of the small bowel, especially in the jejunum. Rarely they may occur in the stomach, large bowel, or rectum. Most cases present in adolescence or early childhood, the commonest symptom being abdominal pain caused by intussusception of the intestine around a polyp. This pain is usually intermittent, but patients may present with an acute abdominal emergency, caused by total obstruction or, as in this patient, infarction of intussuscepted bowel. The polyps frequently bleed and patients may present with recurrent iron deficiency anaemia, rectal bleeding, or melaena. Occasionally bleeding from gastric polyps may cause haematemesis.

The melanin pigmentation is seen as dark brown or grey spots, especially on the lips and inside of the mouth, but it may occur on the face, arms, palms, perianal area, and soles of the feet. The cutaneous pigmentation may fade with age, but the buccal pigmentation persists. Some patients without pigmentation have been described.

Apart from intussusception and bleeding, the other main complication of the Peutz–Jegher Syndrome is an increased incidence of gastrointestinal adenocarcinoma (2–3%), especially in duodenum and proximal jejunum. The polyps themselves are probably not pre-malignant and there have only been two reports of carcinomatous change in hamartomatous polyp. Polyposis of the bladder, nose, and bronchus, is also more common and 5% of female cases have ovarian cysts and tumours.

Management is usually conservative, since there is extensive intestinal involvement. The intussusception often responds to non-surgical measures, but if obstruction fails to resolve or if features of infarction develop, surgery should be performed. When gastro-intestinal bleeding is a problem it may be difficult to identify the polyp(s) responsible for blood loss. Extensive resection should, however, be avoided and with recurrent and troublesome bleeding, arteriography or radiolabelled erythrocyte scanning during the acute bleed may identify the responsible segment, thus allowing a limited resection. The risk of malignant change in the polyps is low.

Multiple polyposis of the small intestine may also occur with Familial Polyposis Coli, Gardner's Syndrome (polyposis coli, osteoma, and soft tissue tumours), Multiple Juvenile Polyposis, Neurofibromatosis, and the Cronkhite–Canada Syndrome. The latter condition is not inherited and consists of multiple polyposis throughout the gastrointestinal tract, alopecia, atrophy of the nails, and increased skin pigmentation. In contrast to the Peutz–Jegher Syndrome, these polyps cause severe diarrhoea with fluid and electrolyte depletion, protein losing enteropathy, and malabsorption.

Case 5

Answers

1. Zollinger–Ellison Syndrome.
2. (a) Gastric acid studies.
   (b) Fasting serum gastrin.
3. (a) Angiography
   (b) Abdominal CT scan.
4. Suggests Multiple Endocrine Adenomatosis (type 1).

Discussion

The most likely diagnosis is the Zollinger–Ellison Syndrome. This disorder was described in 1955 and is characterized by gastric acid hypersecretion, and recurrent upper gastrointestinal ulceration due to non-beta islet cell tumours of the pancreas producing gastrin. It occurs most frequently in the third to sixth decades of life and in 75% of patients a single ulcer is found in the first part of the duodenum. These ulcers respond only partially to standard medical therapy and ulceration recurs after gastric surgery. One-third of patients experience diarrhoea and in 5% of cases this may precede dyspeptic symptoms.

The diagnosis is confirmed by measuring gastric acid secretion and fasting serum gastrin. In 60% of patients basal acid secretion exceeds 10 mmol per hour and is over 60% of maximal acid output, stimulated by either histamine or pentagastrin. In the post-operative stomach, basal acid output over 5 mmol per hour is very suggestive of the Zollinger–Ellison Syndrome. Fasting serum gastrin is elevated in this syndrome but a combination of acid hypersecretion and high serum gastrin may also be found in patients with antral G cell hyperplasia and the 'excluded antrum' syndrome. These conditions may be distinguished by 'provocation' tests. In antral G cell hyperplasia the serum gastrin is markedly increased following ingestion of a protein meal, while in gastrinoma patients, infusion of secretin, glucagon or calcium produces a similar response. In the excluded antrum syndrome none of these stimuli increase serum gastrin.

Once the Zollinger–Ellison Syndrome has been diagnosed, further management depends upon localization of the gastrinoma. These tumours are often small and multiple and 60% not visible at surgery. The two most useful investigations in defining the site of the tumour are arteriography and computerized axial tomography of the pancreas, and these enable localization in 20 – 40% of cases. Recently, transhepatic sampling of portal vein tributaries with measurement of the serum gastrin levels was found to be successful in tumour localization in over 75% of patients. In those where the site of the tumour is unknown or the gastrinoma cannot be completely excised, treatment consists of modifying the target organ response. Most patients may be controlled with high doses of H-2 receptor antagonists, total gastrectomy being reserved for those that show an inadequate response to these drugs.

The presence of hypercalcaemia suggests the diagnosis of multiple endocrine adenomatosis (type 1). This condition is inherited as an autosomal dominant with a high degree of penetrance and adenomata may be found in parathyroids, pancreatic islets, pituitary, thyroid and adrenals. Hyperparathyroidism is found in over 80% of such patients and the Zollinger–Ellison Syndrome in around 50%.

Case 6

Answers

1. (a) Recent weight gain.
    (b) Emepronium bromide tablets.

(c) Smoking.
(d) Alcohol consumption.
(e) Hiatus hernia.
2. Bronchospasm due to aspiration of gastric contents or reflex bronchospasm due to acid reflux into oesophagus.
3. (a) Candida.
(b) Herpes simplex virus.

Discussion

Inflammation of the oesophagus may be caused by the ingestion of corrosive substances, reflux of damaging agents (e.g. acid, pepsin and bile), or infective disorders. Acid reflux is likely to be the main factor in this patient. Many mechanisms help to prevent gastro-oesophageal reflux including the anatomy of the oesophago-gastric junction, the 'squeeze' exerted by the diaphragmatic crura, the effect of pressure on the intra-abdominal portion of the oesophagus, and the mucosal folds of the gastric fundus which may occlude the lumen as intragastric pressure rises. The most important protective mechanism is the lower oesophageal sphincter with its resting tone and ability to adapt quickly to meet changing requirements. However 25% of patients with reflux have normal sphincter pressure illustrating the importance of other mechanisms. Many factors can reduce the lower oesophageal sphincter pressure. Diseases such as scleroderma, neurological and muscular diseases, surgical vagotomy, and alpha-adrenergic antagonists are factors which are not relevant in this patient. Alcohol, smoking and anti-cholinergic drugs like emepronium bromide have the same effect and are relevant in this patient. The presence of a hiatus hernia is very frequently associated with oesophageal reflux and may be relevant in our patient. Some workers have suggested, however, that oesophageal reflux may produce fibrotic shortening of the oesophagus and thus cause a hiatus hernia, so providing an alternative explanation for the association. Obese patients, particularly those who have gained considerable weight in a short time, are prone to develop acid reflux and these features are present in this case. A variety of drugs (e.g. slow release potassium, non-steroidal anti-inflammatory drugs, etc) when lodged in the oesophagus produce local inflammation and mucosal damage and emepronium bromide taken by our patient, is a well known example. If necessary such drugs should be taken standing up with an adequate volume of fluid.

This lady's nocturnal respiratory symptoms are suggestive of acute bronchospasm. Acid or gastric contents refluxing into the oesophagus, through an incompetent lower oesophageal sphincter in the supine position, may enter the bronchial tree causing choking, bronchospasm or even aspiration pneumonia. In addition, recent studies have suggested that acid reflux into the oesophagus may provoke reflex bronchospasm and that some asthmatic attacks may be precipitated by acid entering the oesophagus.

Candida and herpes simplex virus (HSV) are the two commonest oesophageal infections. Other infective agents may affect the oesophagus as part of a generalized infection, but they rarely cause infection limited to the oesophagus. Candida albicans is the commonest fungus causing infection and may be isolated from the mouth (50%) and the stools (90%) of normal individuals. Antibiotics and steroid therapy commonly predispose to such oesophageal infections. Pre-existing oesophageal disease and leucopaenia are other important factors. These patients complain of odynophagia, dysphagia and retrosternal burning. Bleeding and perforation are uncommon and 25% of patients are asymptomatic. The diagnosis is suggested by the endoscopic appearance (white plaques on an erythematous base, oedema, 'cobble-stoning' and ulceration) and is confirmed by the identification of fungal hyphae in biopsy material. Oral Nystatin, 500 000 units 6 hourly, is the treatment of choice but may present difficulties in patients who are unable to swallow liquids. Amphotericin B (0.5 mg/kg/day intravenously) is suggested for such severely affected patients; especially if immunosuppressed. Oral ketoconazole may prove useful in patients who can swallow.

The incidence of HSV oesophagitis is unknown as many cases are diagnosed only at post-mortem examination. It usually occurs in patients with advanced malignancy, immunodeficiency or following trauma, chemotherapy, radiotherapy and steroid treatment. Occasionally it occurs in healthy individuals. Symptoms are similar to those of candida oesophagitis and although the classical endoscopic appearances are of vesicles and later punched out ulcers, it is often difficult to distinguish these from candida oesophagitis. Biopsy, however, reveals eosinophilic intranuclear inclusion bodies and virology may confirm HSV infection. No treatment is usually required but temporary reduction of immunosuppression or steroid therapy is advised, the condition usually settling within a couple of weeks. In severe cases parenteral acyclovir is recommended.

Case 7

Answers

1. Crohn's disease.
2. Erythema Nodosum.
3. (a) Sigmoidoscopy and biopsy.
   (b) Barium enema.
   (c) Barium follow-through.

Discussion

The combination of diarrhoea, conjunctivitis, skin lesions and a high ESR suggest a diagnosis of inflammatory bowel disease. Furthermore, the absence of rectal bleeding and the presence of anal skin tags make Crohn's disease the most likely diagnosis. The skin lesions are typical of erythema nodosum and this is the commonest cutaneous manifestation of inflammatory bowel disease. Other associated skin disorders include pyoderma gangrenosum and psoriasis. The investigations most likely to confirm the diagnosis are sigmoidoscopy and biopsy, barium enema with views of the terminal ileum and barium examination of the small bowel. If these are normal, a colonoscopy with examination of the terminal ileum may detect superficial mucosal disease.

The diagnosis of Crohn's disease depends on the recognition of a pattern of macroscopic and microscopic abnormalities in the gastrointestinal tract. The histological hallmark is the non-caseating granuloma which is found in 60 – 70% of cases, although the frequency of detection depends on the site of origin of biopsy material, amount of tissue available, and diligence of the search. The macroscopic features suggestive of Crohn's disease are discontinuity of the inflammatory process (skip lesions), cleft-like ulcers and fissures (cobblestoning and rose thorn ulcers), fistulae, chronic anal lesions and involvement of the terminal ileum with ulceration and stricture formation (String sign of Cantor). Although it is possible to make a clinical diagnosis from the symptoms, X-rays and macroscopic findings at endoscopy, in most cases a biopsy adds greatly to the diagnostic yield.

In the above patient, Crohn's colitis was confirmed by barium enema and sigmoidoscopy with biopsy. The rectal mucosa, had aphthous ulcers while the enema demonstrated 'skip' lesions in the transverse and descending colon. Granulomas were present in the rectal biopsy. Although the patient made a good initial response to oral steroids and salazopyrine the disease became refractory to medical treatment and necessitated a procto-colectomy 2 years after the initial diagnosis. No evidence of small bowel disease was present on the pre-operative X-rays or at laparotomy.

Case 8

Answers

1. Patterson–Brown–Kelly (Plummer–Vinson) Syndrome.
2. Barium Swallow.
3. Iron deficiency but TIBC is low secondary to hypoproteinaemia.
4. (a) Sjögrens Syndrome.
   (b) Schirmer Test.

Discussion

This patient has the Patterson–Brown–Kelly (Plummer–Vinson) Syndrome, with iron deficiency anaemia, glossitis, koilonychia, and dysphagia at the level of the cricopharynx. The latter is usually due to an oesophageal web, composed of epithelium lying on a connective tissue stroma. Some patients have atrophy of the squamous epithelium at the upper oesophageal sphincter without web formation. Not all patients have anaemia at the time of diagnosis, but have a past history of anaemia. A barium swallow is the best way of demonstrating the post-cricoid web, as endoscopy frequently ruptures the web during intubation and therefore the lesion is not seen. However, it is subsequently important to perform endoscopy with biopsy or brush cytology of the post-cricoid area, because of the development of carcinoma in up to 16% of cases. Treatment comprises correction of the anaemia and relief of dysphagia, the latter being achieved simply by rupture of the web at endoscopy.

The oesophagus may be affected by a congenital web lined by squamous epithelium, and located proximal to the gastro-oesophageal junction. It usually presents with dysphagia in childhood. The oesophagus may also contain other ring-like lesions, the commonest being a Schatzki ring lying at the oesophagogastric junction. The upper surface of this ring is lined by squamous epithelium, and the lower surface by columnar cells. In contrast to the congenital web it rarely causes dysphagia. The diagnosis is confirmed by barium swallow or oesophagoscopy. If symptoms are present these can be controlled by thorough chewing of the food before swallowing. In troublesome cases, pneumatic dilatation or surgical removal of the ring may be performed.

Iron deficiency anaemia is characterized by a low serum iron and high total iron binding capacity, rather than a normal TIBC as in this lady. Her low serum iron and normal TIBC could be attributed to chronic disease, but the clinical signs, blood film, and MCH strongly suggest iron deficiency. Even though iron deficient, this lady's TIBC is not raised because of the hypoproteinaemia (manifested by the low albumin). When there is co-existing hypoproteinaemia, iron deficiency anaemia may be confirmed by finding a low serum ferritin level, which accurately reflects body iron stores.

This patient also has Sjögren's Syndrome which is characterized by xerophthalmia (decreased lacrimation), xerostomia (decreased salivation), and usually, but not invariably, arthritis. This syndrome is an auto-immune condition, and is frequently associated with other auto-immune disorders. The diagnosis may be confirmed by the Schirmer Test, performed by hooking a standardized narrow strip of filter paper, under the lower eyelid, for 5 minutes (see Normal Laboratory Values p. 156). Treatment is concerned with preventing damage to the eyes, and can be achieved by the use of methyl cellulose eye drops.

Case 9

Answers

1. Gallstone 'ileus'.
2. (a) Adhesions from previous surgery.
   (b) External or internal herniae.
   (c) Gallstone ileus.
3. None.

60

Discussion

The patient is suffering from acute small bowel obstruction resulting from impaction of a gall stone in the terminal ileum. The stone is nearly always greater than 2.5 cm in diameter and the condition is particularly common in elderly women. The absence of external herniae and abdominal scars, makes this the most likely cause of small bowel obstruction in patients over the age of 70 years. In a minority of patients the symptoms of obstruction are preceded by an attack of acute cholecystitis; as in the above patient. The gall stone usually enters the bowel through a cholecystoduodenal fistula and impacts in the terminal portion of the ileum, which is the narrowest segment of small intestine. Rarely, the stone enters the colon and lodges in a segment narrowed by sigmoid diverticular disease.

In the present patient no further investigations are necessary to make a definitive diagnosis of gall stone obstruction. The age of the patient, preceding history of acute cholecystitis and features of small intestinal obstruction are highly suggestive of this diagnosis. The presence of a stone in the right iliac fossa, air in the biliary tree and evidence of small intestinal obstruction on the plain abdominal X-rays confirm the diagnosis. In the absence of air in the biliary tree and an obvious stone in the right iliac fossa the diagnosis may be made by performing a barium meal and follow-through examination which will demonstrate a cholecystoduodenal fistula as well as mechanical obstruction of the ileum.

The mortality of gall stone obstruction is about 15 – 20% and this can be attributed to delayed surgical treatment. An emergency laparotomy should be performed and the stone removed through a small enterotomy. Cholecystectomy and closure of the fistula may be indicated if patients develop symptoms of gall bladder disease following recovery from the emergency procedure.

Case 10

Answers

1. Preceding iron deficiency.
2. (a) Small bowel radiology.

(b) Meckel's scan.
(c) Angiography.
3. Angiodysplasia associated with Turner's Syndrome.

Discussion

The microcytic, hypochromic blood film, together with a low serum iron and high TIBC are not consistent with acute blood loss only and suggests the existence of preceding chronic iron deficiency. The most likely explanation is that the acute bleed was preceded by occult gastrointestinal bleeding.

Localizing the source of gastrointestinal bleeding can be surprisingly difficult. The patient's history of melaena suggests that bleeding is occurring proximal to the right side of the colon. Endoscopy has shown no evidence of bleeding proximal to the duodenum or distal to the ileo-caecal valve. Examination of the small bowel for bleeding lesions is thus required, and several tests are available. Radiology of the small bowel may show structural abnormalities such as neoplastic or inflammatory bowel disease, but small lesions are difficult to detect and vascular anomalies may not be visualized. Small bowel enema, with contrast introduced directly into the duodenum through a duodenal tube, is considered by some to be more accurate than the standard small bowel follow-through examination. A radioisotope scan for a Meckel's diverticulum would be indicated in this patient. Fifty per cent of Meckel's diverticula contain ectopic mucosa and two-thirds of these contain gastric mucosa which may ulcerate and bleed. Uptake of technecium 99 by ectopic gastric mucosa demonstrates the presence of such a diverticulum, but does not necessarily imply active bleeding. Angiography can reveal the source of GI bleeding in up to 80% of cases during active haemorrhage. It can demonstrate structural abnormalities and vascular malformations and has the advantage that the active bleeding site may be visualized, but only if bleeding is fairly brisk (greater than 1–1.5 ml/min). Autologous red cells can be labelled with technecium and repeated abdominal scanning over 24 to 48 hours may show accumulation of radioactivity at the bleeding site. Finally, laparotomy with the fashioning of several stomata, and peroperative endoscopy are further steps which may establish a diagnosis. Our patient had a normal barium follow-through examination, negative Meckel's scan and both superior and inferior mesenteric arteriograms showed no lesion. In view of these negative findings laparotomy was performed, and revealed extensive angiodysplasia of the small bowel mainly affecting the serosal surface. Two stomas were fashioned, one in the distal jejunum and one in the terminal ileum. Post-operative bleeding was observed from the proximal stoma. At a second laparotomy an enterotomy was made and peroperative small bowel endoscopy identified the bleeding segment which was excised.

Angiodysplasia most commonly occurs in the right side of the colon but can occur anywhere in the GI tract. It is principally found in the elderly and usually presents as recurrent self-limiting episodes of rectal bleeding often requiring transfusion. There are a variety of morphological types ranging from discrete polypoid angiomata to diffuse capillary haemangiomata but the commonest form is the flat, spider-like ectasia. Diagnosis is difficult especially when lesions are small. Angiography may detect only the larger lesions, but with good bowel preparation and a skilled endoscopist, even small lesions are easily demonstrated at colonoscopy or ileoscopy. If lesions are small and not too numerous, they can be electrocoagulated at the same examination with good results. Alternatively, bowel resection (e.g. right hemicolectomy) may be appropriate. The aetiology of angiodysplasia is unknown. Some have suggested that it represents a hamartomatous process and others an ageing phenomenon. It frequently co-exists with heart disease, especially aortic stenosis. Serosal small bowel angiodysplasia is very unusual but has been described in Turner's syndrome. The reason for this association is unknown.

Case 11

Answers

1. Wilson's Disease.
2. Slit lamp examination of the eyes (Kayser–Fleischer rings).
3. (a) Plasma copper.
   (b) Caeruloplasmin.
   (c) 24 hour urinary copper.
   (d) Liver biopsy.

Discussion

This young patient with a psychiatric history, neurological abnormalities and deranged liver function tests is likely to have Wilson's disease. Clinically this diagnosis would be supported by the presence of Kayser–Fleischer rings (pigment in Descemet's membrane of the cornea) although these have also been described in primary biliary cirrhosis. They appear as a brownish pigment in the lateral and medial aspects of the cornea. Slit lamp examination of the eye may be needed to demonstrate the rings if not clinically apparent. Investigations to confirm Wilson's disease include plasma copper and caeruloplasmin estimations, 24 hour urinary copper and liver biopsy with estimation of liver copper content.

Wilson's disease or hepatolenticular degeneration is an inborn error of metabolism leading to excess tissue copper deposition. It is inherited in an autosomal recessive manner and the incidence is approximately 1/200 000. Copper is excreted mainly by the biliary tract and partially via urine. After absorption copper is transported to the liver and incorporated into copper binding proteins, such as caeruloplasmin. This step is defective in Wilson's disease and hence there is low plasma copper and caeruloplasmin. Copper excretion in bile is also defective. The excess is initially deposited in the liver and then there is 'spill-over' into brain, heart, kidneys and bone. Urinary copper excretion and hepatic copper content is increased. However, there may be some overlap in these biochemical changes with other liver diseases (see Table 1). Urinary copper excretion after a test dose of penicillamine and measurements of radiocopper incorporation into caeruloplasmin may be used in difficult cases. Liver biopsy initially shows some ballooning of cells, fatty change and increase in liver copper concentration. Later fibrosis and frank cirrhosis develop. At this stage portal hypertension with bleeding varices and ascites occur and these may be the presenting symptoms. Other abnormalities seen in more diffuse forms of the disease are osteoporosis, aminoaciduria, and an increased incidence of pigment gallstones (from haemolysis).

Treatment by dietary copper restriction and copper binding agents such as cholestyramine, is ineffective since only trivial negative copper balance is obtained. The most effective therapy is mobilization and removal of body copper stores by chelation. Penicillamine is the most effective agent and the minimum dose necessary to ensure an adequate urinary excretion of copper (>200 μg/24 hours) is employed. Within 2 years the urinary copper excretion returns to below 100 μg/24 hours and it is currently felt that lifelong therapy is indicated. Approximately one-third of patients will develop adverse effects to this therapy. Hypersensitivity reactions such as rashes, arthropathy, lymphadenopathy and marrow suppression occur soon after onset of therapy and are reversible on drug withdrawal. Reintroduction of penicillamine (sometimes under corticosteroid cover) can be achieved without recrudescence of these adverse effects. Early treatment is essential since the untreated condition can be rapidly fatal. Adequate therapy will result in functional recovery of both the hepatic and neurological systems (including the disappearance of Kayser–Fleischer rings).

Table 1: Biochemical changes occuring in Wilson's Disease found also in other liver diseases

	Wilson's disease	*Other liver diseases*
Plasma copper	< 80 μg/ℓ	↑ Chronic active hepatitis (CAH)
Plasma caeruloplasmin	<200 mg/ℓ	↑ Acute hepatitis, CAH
Urinary Cu excretion	>100 μg/24h	↑ Primary biliary cirrhosis (PBC)
Liver copper concentration	>250 μg/G	↑ PBC, CAH
Kayser–Fleischer rings	+	+ in PBC, Chronic cholestasis

Case 12

Answers

1. Achalasia of Cardia.
2. (a) Barium swallow.
   (b) Upper Intestinal Endoscopy.
   (c) Oesophageal Manometry.
3. (a) Hellers Oesophagomyotomy.
   (b) Pneumatic Dilatation.

Discussion

This patient has achalasia of cardia. This is a diffuse disorder of oesophageal motility characterized by absence of peristalsis, a high resting lower oesophageal sphincter pressure, and failure of the sphincter to relax adequately on swallowing. These abnormalities are due to degeneration of ganglion cells in Auerbach's plexus throughout the oesophagus, but the cause is unknown. Infection with Trypanosoma cruzi, which only occurs in South America, causes similar symptoms and abnormalities in oesophageal motility (Chaga's disease).

Low sternal dysphagia, to both liquids and solids, is almost always present in achalasia. In 33% of cases, particularly in the early stages when the oesophagus still has some ability to contract, attacks of retrosternal pain may occur spontaneously or during swallowing. Initially, the dysphagia may be overcome by drinking large volumes of liquid, or by performing a Valsalva manoeuvre. As the oesophagus becomes more dilated, the lower end more tortuous, and the sphincter more fibrous, it becomes increasingly difficult to force food through. As a result regurgitation occurs, particularly after meals and at night, producing aspiration pneumonitis, asthmatic attacks, bronchiectasis or lung abscesses.

In the UK, the three common causes of dysphagia are benign reflux oesophagitis, malignant strictures and motility disorders.

This patient's chest X-ray showed widening of the mediastinum due to oesophageal dilatation. There was no gastric air bubble as fluid in the oesophagus prevents air entering the stomach. There may also be the lung changes listed above. This patient's barium swallow showed a dilated oesophagus with minor non-pulsatile tertiary contractions, and a 'rat-tail' narrowing of the lower end. In the early stages, upper intestinal endoscopy may not detect any abnormality, and the endoscope can quite easily be passed into the stomach. However, when more severe, a dilated and tortuous oesophagus with food residue may be seen and the instrument is difficult to pass into the stomach. Endoscopy is, however, essential to exclude carcinoma which may mimic achalasia, or occur in association with achalasia. Oesophageal cancer is eight times more common in patients with achalasia and usually develops in the middle third of the oesophagus. Oesophageal manometry, the most helpful diagnostic test, shows the features mentioned above.

Treatment with drugs that relax the lower oesophageal sphincter such as nitroglycerine, nifedipine and hydrallazine, has been disappointing. Good results have been obtained in 70–80% of patients with either Heller's oesophagomyotomy, where the muscle fibres of the lower oesophageal sphincter are divided, or by endoscopic pneumatic dilatation to rupture the muscle coat. Unfortunately both procedures predispose the patient to subsequent reflux oesophagitis.

Other important causes of abnormal oesophageal motility include: diffuse spasm, diabetic neuropathy, scleroderma, dystrophia myotonica, myasthenia gravis, and brain stem lesions such as pseudobulbar palsy. They may present with dysphagia or chest pain similar to that of myocardial ischaemia.

Table 2: Clinical evaluation of dysphagia

	Benign Stricture	Malignant Stricture	Achalasia
Prior heartburn	+	−	−
Onset	Gradual	Sudden	Gradual
Progression	Slow and intermittent	Rapid and constant	Slow and intermittent
Dysphagia			
to solids	Early	Early	Early
to liquids	Late	Early	Early
Weight loss	Late	Early	Late

Case 13

Answers

1. (a) Familial Amyloidosis.
   (b) Rectal or jejunal biopsy.
2. (a) Bacterial overgrowth secondary to stasis.
   (b) (i) Jejunal aspiration with anaerobic culture.
       (ii) ^{14}C glycocholate or H_2 breath test.

Discussion

The patient is suffering from familial amyloidosis of the Portuguese type. This rare disorder presents during the third or fourth decade of life and has an autosomal dominant inheritance pattern. The most common manifestations are a sensory or mixed sensory-motor peripheral neuropathy involving the lower limbs and autonomic neuropathy producing intestinal stasis, sphincter disturbances, impotence, postural hypotension, dyshidrosis, and cardiac conduction defects. Physical examination usually reveals features of peripheral or autonomic neuropathy and patients may have irregular or 'scalloped' pupils with an impaired light reflex. Routine haematological or biochemical investigations may reveal evidence of malabsorption. Xylose absorption is markedly reduced and faecal fat output increased in those with intestinal stasis. X-rays of the gastrointestinal tract often show non-specific changes related to steatorrhoea, but may be normal. The diagnosis is obtained by examination of a rectal or jejunal biopsy for amyloid. Although amyloid deposits may be recognized on routine 'H and E' stained biopsy sections, material should be studied using specialized stains such as congo red, crystal violet or thioflavin T. In the above patient excess amyloid deposition was present in rectal and jejunal biopsies and also in gall bladder and appendix obtained at laparotomy 6 months earlier.

In the Portuguese type of hereditary amyloidosis, steatorrhoea is usually due to bacterial overgrowth within the small intestine. Damage to the autonomic nervous system and amyloid infiltration of intestinal smooth muscle lead to decreased propulsive activity and delayed transit time, which in turn cause an increase in the bacterial population of the jejunum and ileum. With massive amyloid deposition pancreatic enzyme secretion may also be reduced and absorption of nutrients across the villous epithelium impaired. In most patients the cause of steatorrhoea can be defined by performing a jejunal aspiration under anaerobic conditions or ^{14}C glycocholate and hydrogen breath tests (see p. 113).

The treatment of all forms of hereditary amyloidosis is very disappointing and mean survival in the Portuguese type is around 1 – 2 years after diagnosis. A variety of cytotoxic drugs, colchicine and prednisolone have been used with little benefit. Death usually results from cardiac arrhythmias or cardiac failure.

Case 14

Answers

1. Ascariasis.
2. (a) Terminal ileum.
   (b) Dispersal of worms without enterotomy.
3. Levamisole, mebendazole or pyrantel.

Discussion

The common causes of intestinal obstruction in a child of this age are intussusception, Hirschsprung's disease, strangulated hernia and obstruction due to a Meckel's diverticulum. All of these diagnoses must be considered. However the preceding history of vague pain, intermittent diarrhoea and weight loss despite a good appetite, suggest a pre-existing abdominal condition. Worm infestation is clearly present as judged by the passage of worms in the stool and the blood eosinophilia. *Ascaris lumbricoides* is one of the commonest parasites infesting man on a worldwide basis. Patients frequently develop a respiratory illness in the early stages of the disease, as this child did, and some months later during the intestinal phase of the infestation, intestinal obstruction may develop, especially in children. Intestinal obstruction due to ascariasis is therefore a likely diagnosis in this child.

Ascaris eggs can survive in moist soil for several years and when viable eggs are ingested they develop into larvae which migrate through the intestinal wall. Passing through the portal venous system and liver they reach the systemic circulation and the lungs. After migration across the alveoli they ascend the trachea and are swallowed and become mature roundworms which attach themselves to the upper small intestine. During migration through the lungs the larvae often provoke a granulomatous reaction with large numbers of eosinophils trying to kill the larvae. Often the early pulmonary phase of the infestation is asymptomatic, but some patients develop mild cough and others a severe Loeffler's Syndrome with pulmonary infiltrates and blood eosinophilia (greater than 10%). If the worm load is low, the intestinal phase is also symptomless although in malnourished children, it may contribute to protein deficiency. Complications of intestinal ascariasis frequently occur in children, the commonest being intestinal obstruction due to the large size of the worms and their tendency to clump together. Biliary ascariasis also occurs and may lead to cholangitis. Other complications include pancreatitis and appendicitis. These complications usually occur because adult worms migrate in response to anaesthesia, fever, and other stimuli and enter small openings like the Ampulla of Vater or the appendix orifice. Two in every thousand infected children between the ages of 1 and 5 years in the USA develop intestinal obstruction. Frequently an abdominal mass is present, worms are passed per rectum and the white cell count is raised. Partial obstruction due to ascariasis may be treated conservatively, but in patients with features of total intestinal obstruction urgent laparotomy is required to confirm the diagnosis and relieve the obstruction. Obstruction usually develops in the terminal ileum where adult worms congregate to form a bolus at the ileo-caecal valve. At laparotomy the worms should be massaged into the caecum avoiding the need for enterotomy but if this is not feasible an enterotomy is performed and the worms carefully removed.

In an uncomplicated case the diagnosis is made by finding eggs, larvae or adult worms in appropriate specimens. Larvae can occasionally be identified in sputum or gastric washings in the pulmonary stage, and eggs can be found in the stools by thick smear and sedimentation during the intestinal phase. One female worm can produce over 2900 eggs/g of faeces! Male worms and immature females produce no eggs and a single brood of females produce only unfertilized eggs, which are difficult to identify in the stool. Suprunova's test for certain volatile fatty acids produced by ascarids and excreted in the patient's urine is often helpful, but immunological tests are of little value. IgM antibodies can be identified but there is cross-reaction with other worm infestations. Ascaris antigen can be injected into the skin as a prick test but although this is a sensitive test it can cause severe reactions and should be avoided. Blood eosinophilia is a useful sign and in the pulmonary phase will often reach 30–50% although in the intestinal phase it is usually around 10%. Barium meal examination may show tubular filling defects and sometimes a white line of barium can be seen within the intestine of a worm! Tubular defects may also be shown in the bile ducts by appropriate contrast studies.

Treatment during the pulmonary phase should be avoided as dying worms often cause more symptoms than live ones. Corticosteroids are very effective in patients with severe pulmonary symptoms. In contrast, intestinal ascariasis should always be treated. Suspected cases should also be treated as it is very difficult to exclude the presence of male worms or immature females. A single dose of piperazine hydrate is effective treatment but newer drugs with lower incidence of hypersensitivity are now available. Levamisole is specific for ascariasis and mebendazole and pyrantel are useful, broad-spectrum antihelminthics for mixed infestations (e.g. hookworm and roundworm). All of these drugs can be given orally as a single dose but this may need to be repeated or the agents given as a 4 day course in heavy infestations. The diagnosis was confirmed in our patient at laparotomy and a bolus of ascarids was dispersed and worms massaged into the caecum. Post-operatively he received a 4 day course of pyrantel.

Case 15

Answers

1. Diverticular disease.
2. (a) Colonic polyp.
   (b) Colonic carcinoma.
   (c) Ischaemic colitis.
   (d) Angiodysplasia.
3. (a) Barium enema.
   (b) Colonoscopy.
4. Diverticulitis.

Discussion

The commonest cause of long standing constipation and abdominal pain in an elderly man is diverticular disease and this was confirmed by a barium enema. Although this disorder may produce rectal bleeding it is important to exclude other causes. About 30% of such patients have another lesion responsible for the haemorrhage, for example, polyps, cancer, angiodysplasia and inflammatory bowel disease (*see* p. 57). Thus colonoscopy as well as radiology may be required to establish the precise diagnosis. Colonoscopy in our patient revealed a 2 cm benign polyp which had not been visible on barium studies.

Colonic diverticula are herniations of mucosa through the muscle layers. The bowel wall of affected areas is thickened and shortened and diverticula develop adjacent to vessels penetrating the muscle layer. The incidence increases with age, with 8% of adults under 60 years and 40% over 70 years having demonstrable diverticula. The sigmoid colon is most commonly involved (95% of cases) and diverticula become progressively less common in the proximal colon. Manometric studies have shown that basal pressures in the colon of such patients do not differ from normal but the response to a variety of stimuli e.g. food, opiates and parasympathomimetics, is increased. These responses may be reduced by opiate antagonists, anticholinergics and smooth muscle relaxants. Cineradiography has shown that the areas most abnormal on manometric examination correspond to the sites of diverticula.

The incidence of diverticular disease is highest in urban areas of developed countries and lowest in rural parts of third world countries. Migrants from these latter areas acquire a similar incidence to the indigenous population within one generation. The pathogenesis of diverticular disease is not known, but present evidence suggests that dietary fibre deficiency may be important. It has been suggested that the low roughage 'Western diet' results in reduction of faecal output and an increase in colonic pressure during colonic evacuation. Exposure of the sigmoid colon to these high pressures over a number of years could lead to the gradual development of diverticula along the points of least resistance in the muscle wall. Increased sigmoid contractions also occur with stress and this factor may be involved in the aetiology of diverticular disease. There are many similarities between the manifestations of this condition and the irritable bowel syndrome and it has been postulated that the colonic motility disturbance results in irritable bowel syndrome during early life and diverticular disease later on.

Most patients are symptomless but extensive disease can result in lower abdominal colic and altered bowel habit, which are thought to be related more to the abnormal motility than to the presence of diverticula. Bleeding may occur from diverticula in the elderly and the exact bleeding site can be difficult to pinpoint. However in 95% of cases the bleeding ceases spontaneously and does not necessitate surgical intervention. The treatment consists of a high fibre diet to increase the faecal residue reaching the distal colon and thus reduce intra-luminal pressures. Therapy with stool bulking agents, such as cellulose or plant residues, may be needed initially but purgatives should be avoided. As with irritable bowel syndrome, smooth muscle relaxants and anticholinergic preparations may provide symptomatic relief (*see* p. 89).

The major complication of this condition (which our patient had) is diverticulitis and this usually results from a localized perforation of a diverticulum. Clinically, the patient develops constant left lower quadrant abdominal pain and fever. The elderly may present atypically with a fever, leucocytosis and raised ESR without much abdominal pain or tenderness. Plain X-rays of the abdomen may show evidence of obstruction but are usually normal. Barium enema examination and colonoscopy are contraindicated during the acute phase of the illness. Treatment is aimed at resting the bowel, relieving obstruction if present and controlling sepsis. Surgery may be required for generalized peritonitis, abscess or fistula formation (to bladder, vagina, skin). When the acute attack resolves, patients should be treated with a high fibre diet which may give symptomatic relief of the abdominal pain and the altered bowel habit.

Case 16

Answers

1. Chronic pancreatitis.
2. (a) Plain abdominal X-ray or ultrasound scan.
   (b) Para-aminobenzoic acid (PABA) test.
3. (a) Late onset cystic fibrosis – sweat test
                                      – sperm count
                                      – scan liver and kidneys for cysts.
   (b) alpha-1-antitrypsin deficiency – measure levels in blood.
4. (a) Correct malabsorption;
   (b) Control Diabetes;
   (c) Alleviate pain.

Discussion

The long standing upper abdominal pain, steatorrhoea, weight loss and diabetes mellitus are indicative of chronic pancreatitis. The presence of pancreatic calcification on a plain abdominal X-ray would confirm the diagnosis. When such calcification is not present ultrasonography, CT scanning, or ERCP can be used to reveal structural pancreatic abnormalities. The PABA test or a more invasive secretory output test will demonstrate functional pancreatic abnormalities (*see* p. 179).

The presence of chronic pulmonary disease, with chronic pancreatitis raises the possibility of 'late onset' cystic fibrosis or alpha-1-antitrypsin deficiency. Cystic fibrosis can be difficult to diagnose in adults since the sweat test has a wider range of normal values than in children. It may be worthwhile measuring sperm counts since oligospermia is common in this disorder. This patient's sperm count and sweat test were normal. In cystic fibrosis cysts may be present in liver and kidneys and therefore ultrasonography and CT scanning of these organs should be performed. Alpha-1-antitrypsin deficiency causes emphysema, but is a rare cause of chronic pancreatitis. The level of this peptide was normal in the above patient (normal 2.0–4.0 g/ℓ).

The commonest known cause of pancreatitis in the UK is alcohol excess. Other important causes include hypercalcaemia, hyperlipidaemia, and haemochromatosis. However, in 50% of cases no cause may be found.

Treatment is aimed at correcting malabsorption, controlling diabetes and alleviating abdominal pain. Pancreatic enzyme supplements (Nutrizym, Cotazym, Pancrex V) are given with meals, and may be combined with an antacid or H-2 antagonist (cimetidine/ranitidine) to prevent inactivation by gastric acid. A low fat diet may be necessary with medium chain triglycerides (MCTs), to boost calorie intake. A diet high in protein and carbohydrate is usually advised. If chronic pancreatitis is alcohol induced abstinence is vital to prevent further damage and to control abdominal pain. Pain is initially controlled with regular analgesics, and 'addictive' narcotics and their derivatives are best avoided. Splanchnic nerve block helps some patients, but results are variable. Pancreatectomy should be considered in patients with intractable pain and when pancreatitis is associated with an obstructed pancreatic duct, ventral pancreas, or pancreatic cyst.

Case 17

Answers

1. (a) Tuberculosis
   (b) Crohn's disease
   (c) Intestinal lymphoma
2. (a) Laparotomy
   (b) Laparoscopy with peritoneal biopsy
   (c) Colonoscopy with ileoscopy.
3. (a) TB – Rifampicin, isoniazid, ethambutol;
   (b) Crohn's – steroids, salazopyrine.
   (c) Lymphoma – cytotoxic drugs, radiotherapy.

Discussion

Ileocaecal tuberculosis

Prior to the development of effective anti-tuberculous therapy, intestinal TB was found in around 80% of postmortem examinations on patients with pulmonary involvement. In countries with effective public health programmes intestinal tuberculosis is rare but in countries such as India the disease has been reported in 5% of unselected postmortems. The ileocaecal region of the gut is most frequently involved and the organism may be either *Myobacterium tuberculosis* or *Mycobacterium bovis*. The symptoms are often non-specific, such as fever, night sweats, anorexia, weight loss and lower abdominal pain and may have been present for several years. Occasionally complications develop such as massive haemorrhage, intestinal obstruction, malabsorption, fistulation or perforation. Physical examination may reveal a fever and in 75% of cases a mass in the right iliac fossa.

Crohn's disease

In contrast to intestinal tuberculosis, Crohn's disease is more common in Northern Europe, where its incidence has increased some 3 to 5 fold over the past 30 years. The ileocaecal region is involved in around 40% of patients and the age at diagnosis is often about 30 years. Abdominal pain is the most common symptom in ileocaecal Crohn's and is usually colicky and located in the right lower quadrant. Other manifestations include anorexia, malaise, weight loss, alteration in bowel habit and peri-anal disease. Extra-intestinal manifestations involving skin, eyes and joints occur in one-third of patients and the intestinal complications include obstruction, malabsorption, occult haemorrhage, fistula formation and perfora-tion. Physical examination may reveal evidence of anaemia and malnutrition, fever, and a right lower quadrant mass.

Primary intestinal lymphoma (*see* p. 106)

Primary lymphoma of the gut is a rare disorder in the UK, the annual incidence being about 1.6/100 000 of the population. In most patients a single segment of ileum or jejunum is involved, but multiple lesions occur in 20 – 25% of cases. Non-specific symptoms, such as anorexia, malaise and weight loss, usually precede localizing symptoms such as abdominal pain. The most common physical signs are abdominal tenderness and a palpable abdominal mass. Fever and hepato-splenomegaly suggest the presence of disseminated disease.

Since the above patient had been resident in India for many years and Crohn's disease occurs less commonly in Asians, the most likely diagnosis is ileocaecal tuberculosis. The presence of fever and splenomegaly are not particularly helpful since these features occur in all the diseases discussed above. The treatment of each condition is quite different and steroids or immunosuppressive drugs, used to treat Crohn's disease and lymphoma, may cause exacerbation and dissemination of tuberculosis. The barium meal and follow-through examination may provide important clues as to the diagnosis but Crohn's disease, ileocaecal TB and terminal ileal lymphoma may occasionally produce similar appearances. Histological diagnosis must, therefore, be obtained. The three ways in which this may be obtained in the above patient are: laparotomy, laparoscopy with peritoneal biopsy and colonoscopy with ileoscopy. Laparotomy will provide the highest yield but the less invasive techniques of laparoscopy with peritoneal biopsy and colonoscopy may also provide definite diagnosis. The biopsy material should also be sent for bacteriological studies and ileocaecal Crohn's will be distinguished from tuberculosis by the absence of caseation and acid fast bacilli on Ziehl–Neelsen staining. Occasionally, in patients considered unsuitable for the above investigations a short trial of anti-tuberculous therapy may help establish the diagnosis. In the above patient a biopsy of the ileocaecal region at laparotomy provided definite diagnosis of ileocaecal tuberculosis.

Steroids and salazopyrine are the most commonly used therapeutic agents for reducing the inflammatory process in Crohn's disease. The value of these and other drugs such as azathioprine and metronidazole are discussed on p. 194. Ileocaecal tuberculosis should be treated with rifampicin, isoniazid and ethambutol for the initial 3 months and isoniazid plus either rifampicin or ethambutol for a further 6 months. A single segment of intestinal lymphoma should be resected, the 5 year survival being around 50–75%. With more extensive disease radiotherapy and chemotherapy are the treatments of choice (*see* p. 107).

Case 18

Answers

1. Solitary rectal ulcer syndrome.
2. (a) Straining.
   (b) Ischaemia.
   (c) Digital trauma.
3. High fibre diet.

Discussion

Several diagnoses must be considered in this patient. A villous adenoma of the rectum often presents as a localized lesion producing mucus, but the histology is not compatible with this diagnosis. Ulcerative proctitis is also a possibility but the lesion is localized and the histology is not consistent with colitis. Irritable bowel syndrome may present with pellety stools and mucus, but the presence of rectal bleeding and the proctoscopic appearance are against this diagnosis. The clinical history and histological features are typical of solitary rectal ulcer syndrome (SRUS).

SRUS occurs equally in men and women, usually in younger patients (peak at 20–29 years). It often occurs in patients who strain at stool and although not rare is frequently unrecognized or misdiagnosed. Many aetiologies have been suggested, including bacterial or viral infection, hamartomatous malformations, or localized inflammatory bowel disease, but there is little definite support for any of these theories. The most likely events involved are prolapse of rectal mucosa during straining at stool with subsequent fibrosis of the submucosa and its blood vessels leading to ischaemic necrosis of the mucosa. Ischaemia of the mucosa could also occur because of impaction of the prolapsed mucosa in the anal canal. Digital trauma may play a small part in the mucosal damage as some of these patients have the habit of introducing a finger into the rectum to aid defaecation, perhaps by reducing a small degree of rectal mucosal prolapse.

The diagnosis of SRUS is based on the clinical features and the histological changes of submucosal fibrosis with smooth muscle fibres passing up between the glands from the muscularis mucosae. Symptoms are very variable, but usually include rectal bleeding and the passage of mucus. Pain though usually mild or non-existent, is occasionally severe. Fifty per cent of patients have a regular bowel habit, the rest being either constipated or having an irregular bowel habit. Ulceration may occur anywhere below the rectosigmoid junction, but is usually located in the lower half of the rectum. The commonest site for ulceration is on the lower anterior or antero-lateral wall. Occasionally there is no ulceration, just an area of apparent proctitis or there may be several ulcers and this may cause confusion in diagnosis.

The treatment of SRUS is mainly symptomatic and aimed at removing the need to strain at stool. High fibre diets and bran are helpful in this respect. Steroid suppositories are often tried but there is no local or systemic therapy that has proved reliably effective. Surgical treatment is only justified when true rectal prolapse is present. Although symptoms can be controlled with the help of these various measures the results of treatment are generally disappointing.

Case 19

Answers

1. Primary biliary cirrhosis.
2. (a) Ultrasound scan to exclude extrahepatic biliary obstruction.
   (b) Antimitochondrial antibody.
   (c) IgM.
   (d) Liver biopsy.
3. Cholestyramine.
4. Serum bilirubin level.

Discussion

This patient has primary biliary cirrhosis, manifesting as generalized pruritis, pigmentation, xanthelasma and a raised alkaline phosphatase. Confirmation of the diagnosis may be obtained from a positive antimitochondrial antibody test, raised serum IgM, normal ultrasound of the liver and biliary tree and typical features on liver biopsy.

Primary biliary cirrhosis is a chronic progressive inflammatory disease occurring in predominantly middle aged females (mean age at diagnosis 60) who present with a slow onset of cholestasis. The aetiology remains obscure, one current hypothesis suggesting that cell mediated immunity is disturbed due to loss of suppressor T cell activity. The disease is characterized by segmental, non-suppurative destruction of bile ducts causing intrahepatic disturbance of bile flow. There is thus cholestasis without large duct obstruction. The initial histological signs include bile duct inflammation, with monocyte and lymphocytic infiltration and non-caseating granulomata. Progression of the disease results in more widespread ductular damage, fibrosis and ultimately cirrhosis.

The usual clinical presentation is persistent pruritus (50–75% of cases) which may precede other hepato-biliary manifestations by several years or may appear for the first time during pregnancy and when taking the contraceptive pill. Pigmentation, xanthoma and hepatosplenomegaly are often present (25%). Portal hypertension with associated bleeding may occur relatively early when the underlying mechanism is often obscure. The earliest biochemical abnormality is a raised alkaline phosphatase (>250 IU/ℓ in 95% of cases) and asymptomatic patients (5%) may be detected during biochemical screening. The serum cholesterol and triglycerides are often elevated and the incidence of gallstones, and a variety of collagen disorders (particularly the sicca and CRST syndromes) and thyroid disease is increased. Prolonged cholestasis may lead to calcium, fat and fat soluble vitamin malabsorption. Bone pain and fractures may occur from a combination of osteoporosis and osteomalacia.

The major serological abnormality is the presence of anti-mitochondrial antibody (95% of patients) but this may be found in other liver disorders (10–20% of patients with chronic active hepatitis). Anti-nuclear and anti-smooth muscle antibodies are seen less frequently (15–35%) and all three major immunoglobulins may be raised, with IgM being the most consistently elevated (85% of cases).

'Non-specific' therapy is directed at correcting nutritional deficiencies (particularly vitamins K and D), and resolving the complications of hepatocellular failure. Pruritus usually responds to cholestyramine which reduces ileal reabsorption of bile salts and thus their accumulation in blood and skin. Immunosuppression with azathioprine and prednisolone have proved ineffective and steroids may exacerbate metabolic bone disease. Since ductular damage leads to accumulation of hepatic copper (80% of this mineral is excreted in bile) penicillamine has been used to treat primary biliary cirrhosis. Although it is effective in reducing the increased liver copper stores, improvement in mortality and morbidity have yet to be shown.

The prognosis of primary biliary cirrhosis is directly related to the serum bilirubin. Many patients run a relatively benign course for many years but the development of a progressive rise in bilirubin level usually heralds the onset of liver failure and death within 2 years.

Case 20

Answers

1. (a) Ischaemic colitis – most likely,
   (b) Ulcerative colitis,
   (c) Crohn's disease.
   (d) Acute diverticular disease,
   (e) Carcinoma of the large bowel,
   (f) Infective Diarrhoea.
2. (a) Barium enema,
   (b) Sigmoidoscopy with rectal biopsy,
   (c) Microscopy and culture of faeces.
3. (a) Gangrene ± perforation,
   (b) Stricture formation.

Discussion

This patient had ischaemic colitis but other conditions considered were ulcerative colitis, Crohn's disease, diverticular disease, carcinoma and infective diarrhoea (particularly, campylobacter and bacillary dysentery). All of these can present with left sided abdominal pain, tenderness, bloody diarrhoea, vomiting, fever, tachycardia and leucocytosis. The clinical features, favouring ischaemic colitis in this patient are a history of post-prandial pain of similar character, and the associated coronary and peripheral arterial disease.

In 70% of cases, ischaemic colitis involves the left colon between the recto-sigmoid junction and the splenic flexure. This area is supplied only by the inferior mesenteric artery (IMA). The rectum rarely becomes ischaemic (5%), because of its dual blood supply from the inferior mesenteric artery and branches of the internal iliac artery. In contrast, the splenic flexure is particularly prone to ischaemia as a result of poor collateral communication between the left colic branch of the IMA and the middle colic branch of the superior mesenteric artery (SMA). The right colon and proximal two-thirds of the transverse colon is supplied by the SMA, and is less commonly affected by ischaemia because of good collateral communications with the coeliac axis. Even when this area of the colon does become ischaemic, following acute SMA occlusion, the associated small bowel ischaemia dominates the clinical picture. In patients over 50 years, ischaemic colitis is most commonly due to atheroma but it can also occur after surgery for an aortic aneurysm, if the IMA is ligated. Diabetes mellitus, hypertension or a hypotensive episode are other predisposing conditions. In the under 50s, the commonest association is with intake of oral contraceptives, although the low oestrogen pill and a policy of not prescribing the pill to women over 35 years, should reduce this complication. Diabetes mellitus is the next most frequent cause (15%) in the younger age group.

The clinical manifestations of ischaemic colitis are very variable and occasionally, inferior mesenteric artery thrombosis occurs without any symptoms or abdominal signs. Over 40% of cases develop the acute form described above while 12% develop gangrenous colitis with shock and peritonitis. Most of the remaining patients present with a history of intermittent abdominal pain (mesenteric angina), rectal bleeding or alteration in bowel habit. As in the above patient, an acute episode may occasionally develop on a background of chronic ischaemia.

Sigmoidoscopy and rectal biopsy are normal in ischaemic colitis but are helpful in excluding the other conditions mentioned. Microscopy and culture of faeces helps exclude infective diarrhoea. A plain abdominal X-ray is not diagnostic but may occasionally demonstrate a narrowed ischaemic segment. The most valuable investigation is a barium enema which, in addition to demonstrating the narrowed area, may show thumb printing and loss of haustrations. Five to ten days after an acute onset, the barium enema may also show mucosal ulceration. Colonoscopy is not indicated in the acute stage when there is a risk of perforating the ischaemic segment. Colonoscopy is useful in those who develop a stricture when carcinoma or Crohn's disease need to be excluded. Selective arteriography is not usually required to confirm the diagnosis of ischaemic colitis.

This man was managed conservatively, with analgesia and blood transfusion. His pain and bloody diarrhoea settled over the next three days. Laparotomy is only indicated if severe bleeding persists or if perforation of gangrenous bowel occurs. If bleeding does not resolve, stricture formation should be considered. Most patients survive acute ischaemic colitis from IMA occlusion, but in SMA occlusion there is a mortality of up to 90%, and those who survive frequently develop nutritional deficiencies from the short bowel syndrome (p. 167).

Case 21

Answers

1. Amoebic colitis.
2. (a) Microscopy of fresh stools, rectal swab or rectal biopsy;
   (b) Serological tests for Entamoeba histolytica.
3. Metronidazole, diloxanide furoate, emetine HC1, tetracycline.

Discussion

The most likely diagnosis is amoebic colitis. Approximately 10% of the world population is infected by *Entamoeba histolytica* and infection is particularly common in tropical and subtropical countries where the standards of personal hygiene and environmental sanitation are low. In some tropical countries as many as 80% of the population are infected and amoebic colitis is a frequent cause of acute diarrhoea with rectal bleeding in travellers returning from such countries. Not all subjects infected with *Entamoeba histolytica* develop dysentery and in studies on human volunteers it has been shown that while most patients who ingest contaminated material become infected, only one-fifth show evidence of colitis. Amoebic liver abscess is a late complication of amoebic colitis and may present many years after the acute diarrhoeal illness. Its presentation is similar to pyogenic liver abscess (*see* p. 47) and treatment is as for amoebic colitis, with aspiration of the abscess being restricted to patients that show an inadequate response.

Entamoeba histolytica exists in 2 forms; the motile trophozoite and the non-motile cyst. The cystic forms are present in the stools of asymptomatic carriers and ingestion of material containing such cysts will result in colonization of the large bowel with amoebae. In the large bowel of carriers, the amoebae browse on the mucosal surface and ingest bacteria and particulate material without invading the epithelium. Some are carried towards the rectum and as the faeces become more solid the amoebae encyst. Once excreted the cysts may remain viable for up to 10 days in a cool and moist environment. If the transit of faecal material along the colon is increased producing diarrhoea, the trophozoites may also appear in the stools. Thus the finding of motile trophozoites in diarrhoeal stools does not necessarily indicate amoebic colitis, and Robert Koch first demonstrated *E. histolytica* in the stools of patients suffering from cholera. The best method of diagnosing amoebic colitis is to demonstrate amoeboid trophozoites containing ingested red blood cells in a fresh stool sample, rectal swab or fresh rectal biopsy. When amoebae invade mucosa they secrete lytic enzymes and ingest red cells from damaged mucosal capillaries. Since trophozoites stop moving when the environmental temperature falls below 37°C, stool samples and biopsy material must be examined within minutes of being collected. In the above patient diagnosis was delayed because only a single, cooled sample was examined. It has been recommended that 3–6 fresh samples should be examined before amoebic colitis can be confidently excluded. Serological tests are occasionally useful in distinguishing amoebic colitis from ulcerative colitis and should always be performed on patients returning from the tropics or subtropics if steroid therapy is contemplated.

Malaise, vomiting, fever and dehydration occur infrequently in amoebic colitis unless patients are immunosuppressed. Steroids cause rapid progression of the disease which may result in gangrene of the colon with signs of severe toxaemia and peritonitis. In the above patient, topical steroid therapy caused a marked exacerbation of the colonic disease and repeat examination of fresh stools at this time confirmed the diagnosis of amoebic colitis.

Metronidazole is the drug of choice in treating amoebic colitis and will usually eradicate infection and relieve symptoms within 5 days (800 mg t.d.s). In some patients organisms may persist and it is now recommended that this drug be combined with diloxanide furoate (500 mg t.d.s), given for 10 days. In severe cases, emetine hydrochloride or tetracycline may help hasten recovery. Infection in asymptomatic carriers is usually eradicated by a 5 day course of metronidazole. Steroid therapy and salazopyrine was discontinued in the above patient and he was given a combination of metronidazole and diloxanide furoate. Diarrhoea and rectal bleeding ceased within 5 days and after 10 days he was well with nearly normal sigmoidoscopic appearances.

Case 22

Answers

1. Bile salt induced (cholereic) diarrhoea.
2. (a) ^{14}C glycocholate breath test.
   (b) Faecal bile salt levels.
3. Cholestyramine.
4. Vitamin B_{12}.

Discussion

The most likely cause of this patient's loose stools is bile salt induced diarrhoea, secondary to terminal ileal resection. Although recurrent Crohn's disease cannot be entirely excluded the absence of other macroscopic disease at laparotomy and the normal barium studies do not support this diagnosis. Significant malabsorption causing diarrhoea is unlikely after such a limited resection.

Ileal resection has many sequelae (*see* p. 166) and interruption of the enterohepatic circulation of bile salts is one of the most important of these. Bile salts are absorbed by the terminal ileum and after passing through the liver are concentrated in the gall bladder. After terminal ileal resection (or dysfunction) unabsorbed bile salts enter the colon where deconjugated dihydroxy bile acids inhibit colonic absorption and stimulate secretion of water and electrolytes and also increase colonic motility. These effects result in watery diarrhoea. Patients present with painless watery diarrhoea which is usually worse after breakfast following the release of large amounts of bile salts stored overnight in the gall bladder. If terminal ileal resection or dysfunction is sufficient to cause malabsorption of vitamin B_{12}, then bile salt malabsorption is invariably present. Normal B_{12} absorption, however, does not exclude bile salt malabsorption. Increased hepatic synthesis can compensate for loss of bile salts but excessive loss eventually leads to a reduction in the circulating bile salt pool. In some circumstances the duodenal concentration of bile salts is insufficient to form adequate micelles and malabsorption of fat occurs. This situation usually develops when more than 100 cm of ileum have been resected. The resultant steatorrhoea tends to be worse later in the day because bile stored overnight in the gall bladder may only prove adequate for absorption of breakfast.

Although bile salt induced diarrhoea is a secretory disorder it does respond to fasting, when gall bladder contraction is prevented.

The ^{14}C glycocholate breath test shows a late rise in exhaled $^{14}CO_2$ but this is difficult to distinguish from the effects of rapid intestinal transit. Increased amounts of radioactively labelled or unlabelled bile salts may also be detected in the faeces in this disorder (see p. 113). Prior to treatment faecal fat estimation is useful to exclude steatorrhoea.

The initial treatment of cholereic diarrhoea should be oral cholestyramine and the response is often used as a diagnostic test for bile salt induced diarrhoea. Cholestyramine is an anion binding resin which is administered as the chloride salt. Bile salts bind to the resin in the jejunal lumen releasing Cl^-ions. The drug is produced as a powder and 4 g in water with breakfast is a reasonable starting dose. Up to 4 doses a day may be necessary. Cholestyramine may bind other drugs and these should therefore be given separately. In renal failure it may cause hyperchloraemic acidosis as the kidney is unable to excrete the absorbed Cl load and if malabsorption is already present cholestyramine, by reducing the uptake of bile salts, will aggravate it. Cholestyramine should not, therefore, be used in patients with ileal resections greater than 100 cm or in the presence of steatorrhoea. Patients with bile salt malabsorption severe enough to cause steatorrhoea should be treated with a low fat diet and medium chain triglyceride supplements (if necessary).

Ileal resection removes the site of vitamin B_{12} absorption and although the above patients' haemoglobin and vitamin B_{12} levels were normal she should be carefully monitored for B_{12} deficiency as this may take several years to develop. Some clinicians advise prophylactic vitamin B_{12} therapy for all patients after terminal ileal resection.

Case 23

Answers

1. Coeliac disease.
2. Jejunal biopsy.
3. (a) Folate deficiency.
   (b) Splenic atrophy.

Discussion

This patient's symptoms, signs and abnormal investigations suggest malabsorption which has led to mineral and vitamin deficiencies. The most likely diagnosis is coeliac disease and this would be confirmed by a jejunal biopsy. In this condition the small intestinal mucosa is damaged after ingestion of gluten containing food. Gluten is found in wheat, rye, barley and malt, but not oats, rice or maize. Coeliac disease occurs predominantly in Western Europe, with the highest incidence on the West coast of Ireland (1 in 500). The incidence in the remainder of Britain is 1 in 2000. There are two peaks of presentation, one between 6 and 12 months of age, and the other between 30 and 50 years. The common manifestations include diarrhoea with steatorrhoea, weight loss, short stature and deficiencies of various minerals and vitamins. In children, failure to thrive is a frequent finding. Other presenting features include oral aphthous ulceration, abdominal distension, weakness, anaemia, nausea and vomiting. Abdominal pain is not a prominent feature. The diarrhoea is often multifactorial resulting from malabsorption, active secretion of fluid and electrolytes by intestinal cells, and secondary pancreatic insufficiency. The anaemia may be due to iron or folate malabsorption and hyposplenism occurs in 30–35% of patients. The mechanism of splenic atrophy in coeliac disease is uncertain but it is thought to be immunologically mediated, possibly through circulating immune complexes. The incidence of coeliac disease is increased some fivefold in the family members of patients and there is an increased incidence of the tissue antigens, HLA-B8, DR 3 and DR 7.

Diagnosis is established from the appearance of total villous atrophy on the jejunal biopsy. The changes are most marked in the duodenum and become less evident distally, probably due to the destructive effect of pancreatic enzymes on gluten. Treatment consists of a gluten free diet for life. Within a month the majority of patients improve subjectively and their jejunal villi start to regrow. It is important not to give a gluten free diet to patients without a pre-treatment biopsy, as many may respond in a non-specific manner or even have a spontaneous remission of symptoms. Appropriate iron, folate, calcium, vitamins and trace elements may need to be replaced. In resistant or critically ill patients corticosteroids often induce a remission. Non-responders may continue to ingest some gluten, often accidently in foods such as some ice creams and gravies. Strict dietary counselling is thus mandatory for patients and their relatives.

Malignant disease of the gastrointestinal tract is the major long term complication of coeliac disease, and there is an increased incidence of small bowel lymphomas (histocytic variety) as well as cancers of the oesophagus and stomach. It is unclear whether a gluten free diet prevents malignant change. Cancers tend to occur in patients over the age of 50 and after many years of malabsorption. The incidence of malignant transformation varies from 0.01 – 10% of patients. Presentation is subacute with clinical deterioration or pain, haemorrhage and perforation. An abdominal CT scan may identify a lymphoma which may be multifocal or diffuse, with associated mesenteric lymph node enlargement.

Case 24

Answers

1. Hepatic adenoma associated with the contraceptive pill.
2. (a) Hepatic scanning (ultrasound/isotope/CT).
   (b) Hepatic angiography.

Discussion

This lady has a benign adenoma of the liver which is associated with intake of the contraceptive pill. Ninety per cent of people with hepatic adenomas are on the contraceptive pill but the incidence of hepatic adenomas in patients on the pill is probably very low. It is more likely to occur in those who have been on the pill for more than five years. Current evidence suggests that oestrogens promote the growth of pre-existing tumours, rather than initiate adenoma formation. In support of this is the fact that people who have never been on the pill may develop hepatic adenomas during pregnancy.

Acute abdominal pain with shock, resulting from bleeding into the tumour or peritoneum, is the mode of presentation in 55% of cases. Chronic abdominal pain occurs in 5–10%, a palpable mass in 10–20%, and 20–40% of cases are asymptomatic, the tumour being found coincidentally at operation for another condition. Hepatic adenomas unrelated to the contraceptive pill are asymptomatic and in 50% are a chance operative finding, reflecting that these tumours rarely create problems without hormone stimulation.

Liver function tests and alpha feto-protein are not helpful in the diagnosis as they are usually normal. If the patient does not require urgent laparotomy, a space occupying lesion can be identified by hepatic isotope or ultrasound scan in 80% of cases. If available, an abdominal CT scan will give an even higher diagnostic yield. Hepatic arteriography is also extremely accurate since the lesions are usually highly vascular and this procedure may be useful when planning subsequent surgery. Although these investigations will not provide histological confirmation, liver biopsy should be avoided in these vascular tumours.

Bleeding from adenomas may be controlled by embolisation of the involved hepatic segment at the time of arteriography. Alternatively, hepatic artery ligation can be performed at laparotomy. A large adenoma causing pain should be resected, if possible. The approach to treatment of uncomplicated tumours is controversial. While some advocate resection, others merely advise discontinuing the contraceptive pill which results in tumour regression. The benign adenoma does not undergo malignant change.

The two commonest hepato-biliary complications of oral contraceptive therapy are an increased incidence of gallstones and intrahepatic cholestasis. Both are caused by the oestrogen component reducing bile secretion and bile flow. Patients with intrahepatic cholestasis present with pruritis and/or jaundice and a high proportion of these suffer from recurrent cholestasis during pregnancy. Contraceptive pills with high oestrogen content rarely cause hepatic vein thrombosis and the Budd–Chiari Syndrome.

Case 25

Answers

1. (a) Irritable bowel syndrome.
   (b) Inflammatory bowel disease.
   (c) Intestinal infection.
2. (a) Stool microscopy and culture.
   (b) Large bowel endoscopy
   (c) Large bowel radiology.

3. (a) High fibre diet.
   (b) Antispasmodic drugs.
   (c) Antidiarrhoeal agents.

Discussion

This patient's symptoms are typical of the irritable bowel syndrome but other disorders that require consideration are inflammatory bowel disease and intestinal infection or infestation. Irritable bowel syndrome is extremely common and affects approximately 15% of the population. It ranks with the common cold as a major cause of industrial absenteeism due to illness and accounts for between one half and two-thirds of patients consulting a doctor because of gastrointestinal symptoms. Although the disorder was originally considered to affect only the colon, there is now evidence that motor activity throughout the gastrointestinal tract may be abnormal and many patients have cardiac symptoms, such as palpitations and dyspnoea, and urinary symptoms, such as frequency and loin pain. The gastrointestinal symptoms are extremely variable even in the same individual. Over 90% of patients have alteration in bowel habit and many experience alternating constipation and diarrhoea. Abdominal pain occurs in 75% of cases and is usually located in the left iliac fossa, peri-umbilical region or left upper quadrant. However, the pain may occur in any portion of the abdomen and may mimic conditions such as appendicitis, gall bladder disease, urinary tract infection and peptic ulcer. Approximately 25% of patients experience painless diarrhoea. Such cases complain of morning diarrhoea ('the morning rush') and are then asymptomatic for the remainder of the day. Although the irritable bowel syndrome may cause severe and debilitating symptoms, the patients are usually well nourished and rarely complain of weight loss. Physical examination reveals abdominal tenderness only and investigations are invariably negative or normal. Occasionally patients with typical features of this syndrome have been found to suffer from Crohn's disease and the presence of weight loss, anaemia, abdominal masses and peri-anal disease should alert the clinician to this possible diagnosis. In patients with a shorter history or exacerbation of symptoms after travel abroad, an infectious disease such as giardiasis, campylobacter enteritis and salmonellosis should be excluded.

There is no 'diagnostic test' for the irritable bowel syndrome. Although abnormalities of colonic motility have been defined, colonic manometry is not routinely available and the results are difficult to interpret. The diagnosis is therefore established by excluding other conditions, in particular inflammatory bowel disease and gastrointestinal infection. The three most useful investigations in the above patient would be stool culture and microscopy, endoscopic examination of the large bowel with biopsy, and radiological studies of the large intestine. In the irritable bowel syndrome, stool cultures are negative. Endoscopy and barium enema examinations may reveal areas of spasm that reproduce the patient's symptoms and are abolished by parenteral anti-cholinergic agents. Occasionally endoscopy reveals large amounts of mucus or melanosis coli if the patient has taken laxatives for long standing constipation.

The management of irritable bowel syndrome is often difficult. A careful explanation of the disorder and how symptoms are produced often relieve the patient's anxiety that there is more serious underlying disease. Any food that produces symptoms, such as fatty foods and cream, should be avoided but there is no consistent food intolerance and no evidence that lactose intolerance occurs more often in this disorder. A high fibre diet may help one-third of patients, particularly those with abdominal pain and constipation. In contrast, those with painless diarrhoea are often helped by an antidiarrhoeal agent, such as loperamide. 'Irritant' laxatives, such as the anthraquinones, should be avoided and constipation treated with a high fibre diet and stool bulking agents. Patients with severe attacks of colicky pain should be given antispasmodic agents such as hyoscine or mebeverine. Sedatives should be reserved for anxious patients or those with persistent symptoms related to unavoidable stress.

Case 26

Answers

1. Pancreatic insufficiency.
2. Vitamin A deficiency.
3. Evidence of nicotinic acid deficiency (Pellagra).

Discussion

This patient's symptoms date from his imprisonment in a South East Asian POW camp and chronic infection or infestation of the GI tract must be excluded. However few organisms persist for over 30 years. Chronic giardial infection may present with steatorrhoea and although amoebiasis can persist for many years it usually presents with colonic diarrhoea. *Strongyloides stercoralis* is a parasite which can persist indefinitely as eggs produced in the gastrointestinal tract can transform to infective larvae within the colon and re-infect the host through colonic mucosa. Severe small bowel infections with this parasite may cause steatorrhoea. Several fresh stools should be examined for organisms, cysts and ova to exclude these various infestations.

The combination of glycosuria and marked steatorrhoea in a well nourished patient strongly suggests pancreatic insufficiency. The temporal relationship between his malnutrition and the onset of diarrhoea suggests a causative link. Prolonged protein deficiency may cause pancreatic atrophy and fibrosis and many individuals develop pancreatic calcification. In our patient, stool culture and microscopy was persistently negative and tests of pancreatic function showed gross pancreatic insufficiency. A CT scan of the upper abdomen showed severe pancreatic atrophy without evidence of calcification.

The cause of this patient's blindness was almost certainly vitamin A deficiency. The daily requirement of this vitamin is 750 μg and it is usually acquired as a preformed vitamin from animal products or as vegetable carotenoid precursors. Large amounts are stored in the liver but low intake eventually leads to deficiency. Initially the patient develops dry eyes (xerophthalmia) and experiences night blindness. Foamy plaque-like lesions called Bitot's spots develop on the temporal side of the conjunctivae. They consist of desquamated keratinised plaques and their foamy appearance is probably due to the presence of gas forming organisms (*Corynebacterium xerosis*). These changes are reversible by treatment with vitamin A. If left untreated irreversible damage occurs to the cornea and lens due to corneal erosions and keratomalacia.

Pellagra (Spanish for 'rough skin') is caused by deficiency of Nicotinic acid (Niacin). Adults require 20 mg daily, either as Niacin or as dietary tryptophan which is converted in the body to niacin. The classical features of pellagra are characterized by the 4 'D's: diarrhoea, dermatitis, dementia and death. Prodromal symptoms include lassitude, weakness and anorexia. The diarrhoea is watery but of small volume and small ulcers may occur in the colon. The skin lesion begins as an erythema, rather like sunburn, but later turns to a dirty brown colour and becomes rough and scaly. The dermatitis is symmetrical and localized to the exposed areas although the face is often spared. The skin lesion is particularly prominent around the neck where it has been dubbed 'Casal's necklace'. Glossitis is common and causes the tongue to appear bright red. Neurological signs are late in onset and include polyneuropathy, coarse tremor and encephalopathy. The prognosis in pellagra is excellent. Oral niacinamide is recommended as it is free from the unpleasant vasomotor effects of nicotinic acid. Improvement is rapid unless irreversible brain damage has occurred.

Water soluble vitamins are not stored in the body in large amounts and therefore clinical deficiency may occur rapidly in the presence of poor nutrition. Thiamine deficiency may be manifest as a chronic progressive sensory-motor neuropathy (dry beri beri) or as high output congestive cardiac failure (wet beri beri). Cerebral syndromes such as Wernicke's encephalopathy are rarely seen in the East, except in Westerners. Diets consisting of polished rice lead to thiamine deficiency since this vitamin is confined to the outer husk. Riboflavin is found with the other B vitamins (pyridoxine, pyridoxal, pyridoxamine) in milk, eggs, fish and meat and deficiency leads to angular stomatitis, glossitis, cheilitis and seborrhoeic dermatitis. Deficiency of vitamin C (ascorbic acid) causes scurvy, characterized in adults by follicular hyperkeratosis with perifollicular haemorrhages, swollen bleeding gums, fatigue and arthralgia. Citrus fruits, milk and other plants are good sources of this vitamin.

The fat soluble vitamins A and D are stored in large amounts in the body and clinical deficiency takes a long time to develop. Vitamin K is not stored in large amounts and deficiency occurs more readily.

Case 27

Answers

1. Haemochromatosis.
2. (a) Serum iron and total iron binding capacity.
   (b) Serum ferritin.
   (c) Liver biopsy.
3. Regular venesection.

Discussion

This patient has haemochromatosis and presents with diabetes, arthritis and hypopituitarism. This diagnosis would be supported by finding a raised serum iron with low TIBC and a raised plasma ferritin (often 10–20 times the normal upper limit). If available, a CT scan is said to show increased hepatic tissue density from excess iron deposition. To confirm haemochromatosis a liver biopsy is required. This will demonstrate a large increase in stored iron in hepatocytes and may show histological changes ranging from fibrosis through to a frank cirrhosis. Excess iron deposition also occurs in the pancreas, heart and pituitary gland leading to functional impairment of these organs. Other clinical features include a non-specific arthropathy affecting large joints (with calcification of the articular cartilage), persistent fever and generalized pigmentation (bronze diabetes).

The prevalence of haemochromatosis is 1–2/10 000 and there is an association with the A3 and B14 HLA antigens. Twelve per cent of siblings are affected and it may be detected in the asymptomatic phase during screening of the family of an affected patient. Present evidence suggests that iron absorption in these patients (usually only about 10% of ingested iron) increases inappropriately although the exact mechanism of this is unclear. The sex ratio is 5:1 (M:F). Men present usually after the age of 40 and women develop manifestations 10–20 years later because of the iron loss during menstruation. There is an increased risk of hepatoma (30–40% of patients) particularly in those patients who have developed cirrhosis.

Haemochromatosis must be distinguished from haemosiderosis, where excess iron storage occurs (e.g. multiple transfusions) without parenchymal damage. Early diagnosis and treatment appears to improve longevity and delay complications, and all relatives should be screened by clinical examination together with estimation of liver function tests and serum ferritin. If abnormalities are detected, then a liver biopsy is indicated. The major differential diagnosis is alcoholic liver disease where iron ingestion, usually in beer, is increased. In this condition, however, the serum ferritin is modestly raised and there is only a slight increase in hepatic iron.

The treatment of choice is venesection of 500 ml (250 mg iron) once or twice weekly. The average patient has 20–40 grams of excess stored iron and treatment needs to be continued until serum ferritin and iron are within the normal range. Desferrioxamine is of little value in this condition as the amount of iron that it chelates is insignificant (20 mg/day). Treatment improves established damage such as diabetes, testicular atrophy, cardiomyopathy and arthropathy, but specific therapy for these complications may also be required (e.g. insulin and testosterone). Serum ferritin should be measured at 3 monthly intervals after the initial treatment course and venesection performed when values become elevated. Prognosis depends on whether cirrhosis is established before the diagnosis is made. The risk of hepatoma is not diminished by therapy although there is some evidence that all the complications, including hepatomas, can be avoided if therapy is initiated in the pre-cirrhotic stage.

Case 28

Answers

1. Gilbert's Syndrome.
2. (a) Levels of unconjugated bilirubin.
   (b) Reticulocyte count.
   (c) Fasting serum bile acids.
3. Reassurance.

Discussion

The most likely diagnosis is Gilbert's Syndrome. Chronic hepatitis is less likely as this is usually associated with elevated transaminases. Gilbert's Syndrome is often detected fortuitously, or because an episode of viral hepatitis is 'slow to resolve'. Gilbert's Syndrome is thought to arise from impaired activity of glucuronyl transferase, although in some instances there may be defective uptake of organic ions from blood into hepatocytes. The jaundice is not manifest before puberty and the bilirubin levels become significantly higher in males than in females. There may be three genetically distinct subtypes; all with dominant inheritance. Over half the patients complain of episodic malaise, fatigue, and non-specific gastrointestinal symptoms. Jaundice is usually mild and often missed by the patient until it becomes more marked following viral hepatitis, fasting, a febrile illness, excess alcohol, menstruation, or pregnancy.

The diagnosis should only be made if there is unconjugated hyperbilirubinaemia of 6 months duration, in the absence of haemolysis and if there is no other clinical or biochemical evidence of liver disease. This patient's unconjugated bilirubin was 40 μmol/ℓ out of a total of 50 μmol/ℓ. When total levels of bilirubin are only slightly elevated, however, the technique for measuring unconjugated bilirubin is inaccurate and therefore some centres prefer measuring fasting serum bile acids, which are always normal in Gilbert's syndrome and elevated in most liver diseases. It is rare for the bilirubin level to be greater than 100 μmol/ℓ in a healthy person with Gilbert's syndrome. If the above criteria are fulfilled, and there is no reason to suspect chronic liver disease, there is no need for further investigation. However, if in doubt, further supportive evidence may be obtained from challenge tests. Hyperbilirubinaemia can be enhanced by fasting (400 Kcal/day for 3 days); by giving a carbohydrate load; or by slow I/V injection of 50 mg nicotinic acid. A liver biopsy is rarely indicated in Gilbert's Syndrome and if performed, will show a normal liver. Delayed excretion of cholangiographic contrast medium may result in a mistaken diagnosis of gall bladder disease. Usually no therapy is needed but if the jaundice is sufficient to cause cosmetic problems, up to 60 mg t.d.s of phenobarbitone will promote uptake into, and storage of bilirubin in the liver. Life span is normal.

Hereditary hyperbilirubinaemia also occurs in Crigler–Najjar and Dubin–Johnson Syndromes. The Crigler–Najjar Syndrome has two distinct forms. Type I is inherited as an autosomal recessive gene and results from complete absence of hepatic glucuronyl transferase activity. Severe jaundice develops within a few hours of birth, kernicterus supervenes in 75% of cases and death usually occurs within a few months. Other liver function tests and liver histology are normal. The Type II form may be inherited as an autosomal dominant, or it may be due to homozygosity for genes which in heterozygotes produce at least some cases of Gilbert's syndrome. It is associated with reduced hepatic glucuronyl transferase activity. Jaundice usually develops in the first year of life, but may be as late as early adulthood. Jaundice is increased by the same factors mentioned in Gilbert's syndrome. Again liver function tests and histology are normal. The jaundice in Type II, in contrast to Type I, can be improved with phenobarbitone therapy and the prognosis improved.

Dubin–Johnson Syndrome is inherited as an autosomal recessive gene. In contrast to Gilbert's syndrome and Crigler–Najjar syndrome, the hyperbilirubinaemia is predominantly conjugated due to an inability to excrete conjugated bilirubin into bile. Patients usually present in adolescence or early adulthood with jaundice, malaise, and abdominal discomfort. Pregnancy and oral contraceptive drugs, which impair hepatic excretion of bile, aggravate the jaundice. Routine liver function tests are normal and liver biopsy shows diagnostic dark brown or black pigment granules in the hepatocytes and Kupffer cells. The bromsulphthalein test is also diagnostic showing normal clearance at 45 minutes, but raised levels at 90 and 120 minutes. Hepatic excretion of other organic anions is also affected and the gall bladder cannot be visualized radiologically.

Case 29

Answers

1. Osmotic diarrhoea.
2. Lactose intolerance.
3. (a) Jejunal biopsy + enzyme estimation.
   (b) Hydrogen breath test.
   (c) Lactose tolerance test.
4. Increases delivery of lactose to small bowel.

Discussion

The stool studies indicate the presence of an osmotic diarrhoea. Normal faecal weight in the UK is less than 200 g and thus a stool weight of 500 g confirms the existence of water malabsorption or secretion by the gut. The stool osmolality is high (normal less than 350 mosmol/kg) and there is a marked gap between the measured osmolality (430) and calculated osmolality (twice the sum of Na^+ and K^+: 302). This discrepancy is due to a solute present in the stools and stool weight decreases markedly during a period of fasting. A further abnormality is the low stool pH and this strongly suggests a diagnosis of lactose intolerance.

Lactose intolerance is the most common type of carbohydrate malabsorption and is present in 3 – 20% of North European and

North American white adults. Some populations such as North American Indians and negroes, Asians and various African tribes have a very high prevalence of this disorder (70–95%). The majority of such individuals develop lactase deficiency after the first 6 months of life and congenital deficiency of the enzyme is rare. Decreased activity of lactase and other disaccharidases may also occur secondary to other mucosal diseases such as coeliac disease, gastroenteritis and Crohn's disease. In most mammals, intestinal lactase activity decreases rapidly after weaning and a similar response occurs in those populations with a high incidence of lactose intolerance. Whites of European origin retain lactase activity into adulthood and it is possible that this reflects milk drinking patterns in earlier generations that led to selective survival of those capable of using milk as a source of nutrition.

Although the history and stool analysis strongly suggest a diagnosis of lactase deficiency, three tests are routinely used to confirm lactose intolerance. The most accurate test involves the measurement of disaccharidase activity in intestinal mucosa obtained by peroral jejunal biopsy. Histological examination of the specimen also enables the exclusion of disorders causing secondary lactase deficiency. An accurate, non-invasive test of lactose intolerance is the hydrogen breath test. Subjects ingest 50 g of lactose and the hydrogen content of breath samples is measured at 10 minute intervals for 4 hours.

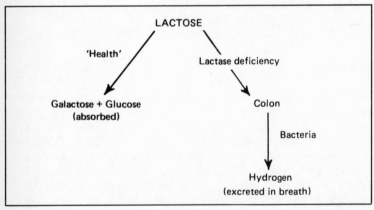

Figure 1

Healthy subjects excrete small amounts of hydrogen in the breath and this is not increased by lactose ingestion. In lactose deficiency, lactose is malabsorbed and is metabolized by colonic bacteria resulting in substantial increases in breath hydrogen. The lactose tolerance test was once used to diagnose this condition but is considerably less accurate and may be abnormal in up to 30% of healthy subjects.

In some individuals lactose intolerance remains latent until the delivery of lactose to the small intestine is substantially increased. This may result from increased milk consumption (main dietary source of lactose) or more rapid gastric emptying (following gastric surgery). Occasionally, surgery results in very rapid emptying of lactose that may overwhelm even normal lactase activity. The colon is capable of salvaging a considerable amount of malabsorbed lactose and this may explain the latency of the condition in some subjects. Thus the development of diarrhoea after partial or total colectomy may also be due to the 'unmasking' of latent lactose intolerance.

Case 30

Answers

1. The patient has a secretory diarrhoea.
2. (a) Stool microscopy and culture.
   (b) Serum gut hormone profile (VIP, gastrin, calcitonin).
   (c) Laxative screen.
3. (a) Correct acidosis, fluid and electrolyte deficiencies.
   (b) Lower serum calcium.

Discussion

The stool electrolyte results reveal that the sum of Na^+ and K^+ with their respective anions, account entirely for stool osmolality (i.e. $(Na+K) \times 2 =$ Osmolality) confirming that the patient has a secretory diarrhoea. Although there are many causes of secretory diarrhoea most are due to acute enteric infections which are self limiting. Chronic secretory diarrhoeas may be due to infections like giardiasis, surreptitious laxative abuse or a hormone producing tumour. The time course of the diarrhoeal illness in this patient suggests a chronic secretory diarrhoea.

Infective causes especially giardiasis should be excluded by repeated microscopic examination and culture of faeces and microscopy of jejunal aspirate. The hormonal causes of secretory diarrhoeas include the Verner–Morrison Syndrome (VIP producing tumour), Zollinger–Ellison Syndrome (*see* p. 135), carcinoid tumours (*see* p. 135) and medullary carcinoma of the thyroid which produces both calcitonin and prostaglandins. Useful tests include a hormonal profile measuring serum gastrin, vasoactive intestinal polypeptide (VIP) and calcitonin. Urine should be sent for hydroxyindole acetic acid estimation (5 HIAA). Since hormone secretion may vary, several estimations should be performed. This patient's clinical history strongly suggests a hormone producing tumour and indeed hypercalcaemia, unrelated to hyperparathyroidism, is a common feature of such tumours (*see* p. 97).

Regardless of the diagnosis, proper management of this patient begins with correction of acidosis and fluid and electrolyte deficiencies. Serum calcium should be promptly lowered by appropriate means (e.g. IV phosphate). After these initial measures further studies may be performed to localize the tumour and delineate metastases, and attempts made to reduce hormone output from the tumour or to counteract their secretory effects.

Investigation of this patient revealed raised serum VIP and metastatic deposits in the liver (on ultrasound scan). Most VIP producing tumours occur in the body or tail of the pancreas and 30% are malignant with metastases at the time of presentation. Patients present with severe watery diarrhoea although this may be episodic. If a vipoma can be identified, the treatment of choice is subtotal pancreatectomy. If there is no evidence of spread, blind subtotal pancreatectomy is probably justified. Palliative treatment only is indicated when metastases are present. Opiates, phenothiazines and lithium all have antisecretory effects, and oral glucose-electrolyte solutions stimulate absorption helping to maintain hydration although not reducing stool output. Cytotoxic therapy (e.g. streptozotocin) may reduce hormone output, as may embolization of liver metastases.

In our patient no pancreatic lesion was identified by ultrasound or CT scanning. Embolization of the liver metastases and a course of streptozotocin and 5 fluoro-uracil caused a temporary reduction in stool output as did lithium therapy. Despite these treatments the patient died 4 months later and post-mortem examination revealed a small malignant vipoma in the tail of the pancreas with metastases in the liver and spine.

Case 31

Answers

1. (a) Crohn's disease.
   (b) Radiation enteritis.
2. (a) Colonoscopy with biopsy.
   (b) Barium follow-through.

Discussion

This patient has malabsorption suggesting small bowel disease, a caecal stricture and an abnormal rectum. The most likely diagnoses are radiation enteritis and Crohn's disease. A colonoscopy with biopsy of the caecal stricture is of value since it may distinguish between these two conditions and exclude other causes of a caecal stricture such as tuberculosis and carcinoma (neither of which could adequately explain the above clinical picture). Barium follow-through examination would also help define any areas of small bowel involved. Colonoscopy in the above patient revealed changes of radiation colitis.

The incidence of radiation enteritis is dose related. Overall, 8% of patients given radiotherapy to the abdomen develop symptoms. Radiation damage to the gastrointestinal tract is either acute or chronic and can affect small or large bowel. Acute exposure leads to a self-limiting illness with nausea, vomiting and diarrhoea lasting a few weeks after completion of treatment. A symptomatic colitis can occur immediately after radical radiotherapy to the pelvic organs resulting in tenesmus, diarrhoea with mucus and occasionally rectal bleeding. A sigmoidoscopy will show oedematous inflamed mucosa with loss of vascular pattern and multiple bleeding points. The more chronic form may develop from months to many years after irradiation and usually follows extensive radiotherapy for pelvic malignancy. Previous surgery or pelvic inflammatory disease increase the risk of bowel problems since loops of intestine may be fixed by adhesions and continuously exposed to radiation. Small intestinal involvement may result in a stricture causing intestinal obstruction, malabsorption from mesenteric lymphatic fibrosis or necrosis and perforation of a segment of bowel. Fistulae between loops of bowel may also occur. In the colon the recto-sigmoid area is most commonly affected. The mucosa may be haemorrhagic or after healing appear atrophic with numerous telangiectasia. In the right colon, these telangiectasia are similar to those found in forms of acquired angiodysplasia. Histology of the acute lesion shows an intense acute inflammatory response. In the chronic form there is an arteritis with submucosal fibrosis and lymphatic obstruction. If the proximal gut is affected a jejunal biopsy may show abnormal villous architecture.

Medical management of these patients is often difficult. Symptomatic treatment with nutritional supplements and a low residue diet may be helpful. Cholestyramine or opiates may help control diarrhoea and some patients respond to prostaglandin synthetase inhibitors, such as indomethacin. Surgery is associated with a high morbidity and healing is poor with substantial risk of anastomotic leakage. Long term prognosis is unpredictable but often poor once symptoms become established or progressive.

Case 32

Answers

1. It indicates the presence of pre-sinusoidal portal hypertension.
2. Portal vein thrombosis secondary to biliary tract surgery and septicaemia.
3. Acute onset of portal vein thrombosis.
4. Trans-splenic portography or superior mesenteric angiography.

Discussion

This man has portal hypertension resulting in oesophageal varices and splenomegaly. Portal hypertension is usually due to increased portal venous resistance and this may originate either within the extrahepatic or intrahepatic vessels.

It is unlikely that he has cirrhosis since there are no stigmata of chronic liver disease, and liver function tests are normal. The past history of a transected bile duct and subsequent septicaemia suggests that the extrahepatic portal hypertension has resulted from portal vewin thrombosis. The normal wedged hepatic venous

Table 3: Causes of portal hypertension

Extrahepatic (Always Presinusoidal)	Presinusoidal	Intrahepatic Postsinusoidal	Mixed
50% idiopathic	UK Congenital hepatic fibrosis Myelofibrosis Chronic myeloid leukaemia Hodgkins disease Sarcoidosis Arsenic Rx for syphilis Polyvinyl chloride exposure	Budd–Chiari Syndrome	Cirrhosis (Commonest cause of portal hypertension in UK)
Children Umbilical infections Umbilical catheterization Infection – dehydration – thrombosis			
Adults Tumour Invasion Infection – peritonitis – septicaemia Biliary Tract Surgery	Worldwide Schistosomiasis –		

Table 4: Presenting features of portal vein thrombosis

'Acute' onset	'Chronic' onset	
Transient ascites	Bleeding oesophageal varices	(50%)
	Splenomegaly	(17%)
	Ascites	(12%)

pressure (WHVP) confirms presinusoidal portal hypertension. The WHVP is performed by passing a catheter percutaneously, usually via the femoral vein, into the hepatic vein, where it is wedged in a small branch, and the pressure measured. The normal WHVP is less than 5 mmHg. Patients with cirrhosis causing mixed intrahepatic portal hypertension usually have a WHVP elevated above 10 mmHg.

The various causes of portal hypertension are summarized in Table 3.

Regardless of whether the onset is acute or chronic, 20% of adults with portal vein thrombosis have ascites and 40% hepatic encephalopathy, at some stage. Both of these are poor prognostic features.

When extrahepatic portal vein obstruction is suspected, supportive evidence can be derived from failure to visualize a patent portal vein with grey scale ultrasonography or by finding a normal wedged hepatic venous pressure. Definitive proof is obtained by the inability to outline a complete portal venous system during superior mesenteric angiography or trans-splenic portography.

Management of ascites and encephalopathy is as in cirrhosis (*see* p. 174). However, in contrast, haemorrhage from oesophageal varices in pre-sinusoidal portal hypertension can often be managed conservatively. At present, endoscopic sclerotherapy appears to be the initial treatment of choice and emergency surgery is reserved for bleeding which is life-threatening or not controlled by medical measures. Oesophageal transection is currently the operation of choice. If recurrent bleeding occurs, splenorenal or mesocaval shunt operations appear to be the most effective. In Webb and Sherlock's series patients managed medically did not die from haemorrhage and had a longer survival from diagnosis (33 years compared with 19 years in the operated group).

Case 33

Answers

1. (a) Drug intake.
   (b) Alcohol consumption.

2. (a) Chronic liver disease.
   (b) Felty's syndrome.
   (c) Amyloidosis.
3. (a) Stabilize circulation.
   (b) Detect cause of bleeding.

Discussion

The items of information that would be most helpful are a history of heavy alcohol consumption and intake of drugs which damage the gastric mucosa. A variety of non-steroidal anti-inflammatory drugs and steroids are used to treat rheumatoid arthritis and these have been shown to damage gastric mucosa and lead to upper gastro-intestinal bleeding. Chronic alcohol ingestion may cause gastro-intestinal haemorrhage from several sources. Alcohol damages gastric mucosa and some patients bleed from gastritis or gastro-duodenal ulceration. Vomiting after the consumption of large amounts of alcohol may cause a Mallory–Weiss tear with subsequent bleeding. Finally, alcoholic cirrhosis leads to the development of oesophageal varices and these may cause massive haemorrhage.

The splenomegaly may be caused by chronic liver disease, Felty's syndrome or amyloidosis complicating long standing rheumatoid arthritis. The presence of marked proteinuria would support the latter diagnosis and this could be confirmed by staining a rectal biopsy for amyloid (*see* p. 67). The main priorities in the initial management of this patient include: appropriate replacement of the blood volume deficit with careful monitoring of the pulse, blood pressure and central venous pressure, possibly nasogastric aspiration to detect evidence of continued bleeding or rebleeding, and diagnosis of the cause of haemorrhage. Upper gastrointestinal endoscopy is superior to radiology in diagnosing the cause of haemorrhage and should be performed when the patient is haemodynamically stable. Large quantities of blood and clots may be removed if necessary by means of ice cold saline lavages performed immediately prior to endoscopic examination. In the above patient, endoscopy revealed diffuse gastritis with 3 discrete antral ulcers, which were benign on histological and cytological examination. The patient had been regularly taking 3 g of aspirin per day for her joint symptoms and this was considered to be the cause of the gastric mucosal damage.

Severe upper gastrointestinal bleeding accounts for approximately 25 000 hospital admissions and around 2000 deaths per year in the UK. The major cause of bleeding is peptic ulcer disease, variceal bleeding and malignancy accounting for only 5–6% of the total. The role played by drugs in the pathogenesis of upper gastrointestinal haemorrhage remains controversial and most of the well controlled studies have only examined aspirin. There is considerable evidence showing increased aspirin consumption in patients with upper gastrointestinal bleeding compared with matched controls, but whether this reflects a cause and effect relationship remains to be established. A recent Nottingham study has shown increased paracetamol intake in such patients, and the authors suggest that up to one-third of patients with gastrointestinal bleeding may take analgesics for the symptoms of haemorrhage. The Boston Collaborative Drug Surveillance Programme published results in 1974 which showed that gastrointestinal haemorrhage was only associated with heavy and prolonged aspirin use, and predicted that only 15/100 000 such users would be admitted to hospital per year with this complication. Apart from numerous anecdotal reports there is little scientific evidence that other non-steroidal drugs or steroids actually cause gastrointestinal bleeding. While acute exposure of the stomach to such drugs results in mucosal damage there is increasing evidence that the stomach adapts and the mucosa returns to normal with chronic ingestion of these drugs. Patients with rheumatoid arthritis have a higher incidence of peptic ulcer disease, regardless of drug intake, and it has not been established that treatment with steroids or non-steroidal anti-inflammatory drugs increases the incidence of either gastric or duodenal ulcer in these patients. In patients taking large amounts of aspirin over prolonged periods the risk of developing gastric ulcer is quite low (Boston study: 10/10 000 heavy users per year).

Case 34

Answers

1. (a) Decreased intake of iron and folate.
   (b) Malabsorption of Iron and Vitamin B_{12}.
   (c) Blood loss.

2. (a) Blood film.
   (b) Serum iron and TIBC.
   (c) Serum B_{12} and folate.
   (d) Gastroscopy.

Discussion

Reduced intake of food due to a small gastric remnant may contribute to anaemia after gastrectomy. Up to 53% of such patients become anaemic and iron, B_{12} and folate deficiency may occur. Iron deficiency is the commonest and may be due to a number of factors, such as decreased intake of iron, chronic blood loss from gastritis or stomal ulceration, and malabsorption of iron due to lack of gastric acid. Vitamin B_{12} malabsorption is mainly due to loss of intrinsic factor but bacterial overgrowth in the small bowel may also play a part. Folate deficiency is mainly due to inadequate intake. Recurrent gastric ulcer is very unlikely after 20 years, but carcinoma arising in the gastric remnant is well described (see below) and would explain the weight loss and anaemia. Tuberculosis is more common in postgastrectomy patients and other unrelated causes of anaemia such as blood loss from the lower gastrointestinal tract must also be considered.

The type of anaemia must be defined by blood film and serum levels of iron, vitamin, B_{12}, and folate. Weight loss and anaemia in a post gastrectomy patient makes investigation of the gastric remnant essential. Barium meal may reveal stomal ulceration or a gastric stump carcinoma, but endoscopy is more accurate in the post operative stomach and has the added advantage of providing biopsies. In this patient, the anaemia was due to mixed iron and B_{12} deficiency and gastroscopy revealed a small polypoid carcinoma near to the anastomotic site.

Gastric carcinoma occurs most commonly in males over the age of 45 years. Smokers and patients with blood group A have an increased risk. Other unknown genetic and environmental factors must operate because gastric carcinoma is particularly common in Japan and very uncommon in rural Africa. Although no polyp-cancer sequence has been identified in the stomach, benign gastric polyps are found in 10% of patients with gastric carcinoma and some authorities consider them to be premalignant especially when large (>2 cm) or when associated with achlorhydria. Benign polyps are more common in patients with pernicious anaemia, who also have a high incidence of chronic atrophic gastritis, and when followed for 15 years after diagnosis have a 10–20 fold increased risk of developing gastric carcinoma (which is not prevented by B_{12} therapy). Chronic atrophic gastritis per se is considered a premalignant condition and is present in most patients with pernicious anaemia and 80% of patients with gastric carcinoma. Chronic atrophic gastritis is common however in the elderly and some workers believe it to be an ageing phenomenon. Gastric surgery may predispose to carcinoma of the stomach although the evidence is conflicting. Some authors note an increased incidence after operation for benign gastric ulcer or duodenal ulcer, particularly when gastroenterostomy has been performed. Gastric carcinoma occurs in up to 3% of patients 15 years after partial gastrectomy, and usually occurs near the anastomosis where chronic atrophic gastritis is common, possibly from reflux of bile and pancreatic juice.

Hypertrophic gastritis (Menetrier's disease) is an uncommon condition which is also thought to be premalignant. It may present with epigastric pain or vomiting, and is characterized by large tortuous folds seen on barium examination or at endoscopy. Biopsies show hyperplastic mucus-producing glands replacing the normal architecture and this usually results in hypochlorhydria. Protein loss may occur from the mucosa and indeed protein losing enteropathy was first described in a case of Menetrier's disease. Treatment is symptomatic with antacids and a high protein diet. Partial gastrectomy should be reserved for those with disabling symptoms.

Case 35

Answers

1. (a) Small bowel lymphoma.
   (b) Crohn's disease.
2. (a) Jejunal biopsy.
   (b) Ultrasound, CT scan of the abdomen.

Discussion

A young patient with a short history of a malabsorption, and an abdominal mass could have Crohn's disease or a small bowel lymphoma. A jejunal biopsy may identify a proximal lymphoma or jejunal involvement with Crohn's disease. An ultrasound or CT scan of the abdomen may identify an abdominal abscess associated with Crohn's disease or enlarged abdominal lymph glands caused by a lymphoma. In the above patient, jejunal biopsy confirmed the presence of a lymphoma.

Primary gastrointestinal lymphomas are usually of the non-Hodgkin's variety and the UK annual incidence is around 1.6 per 100 000 of the population. Primary Hodgkin's disease of the gut has decreased in incidence over the last few decades and is now a rare cause of intestinal lymphoma.

Lymphomas may be localized to one segment of intestine or diffuse and comprise 12 – 18 per cent of small bowel malignancies. A variety of histological types have been described, for example diffuse histiocytic, poorly differentiated lymphocytic and inter-mediate differentiated lymphocytic, and each has its own malignant potential and pattern of spread. In addition, lymphoma may compli-cate pre-existing coeliac disease or dermatitis herpetiformis when the cell type is histiocytic. Rare types of primary intestinal lym-phoma include Mediterranean lymphoma and α-chain disease. Both of these have a particular geographical distribution and it seems likely that α-chain disease is a variant of Mediterranean lym-phoma with excessive production of IgA heavy or α chains.

The age of presentation exhibits a bimodal distribution with peak frequencies in the second decade and around the fifth and sixth decades. The male to female ratio is 2:1 and common manifestations include marked weight loss, abdominal pain and diarrhoea. A pyrexia occurs in around half of all cases and an abdominal mass in 25 – 50 per cent. Other clinical features include finger clubbing, intestinal bleeding, obstruction, perforation and intussusception. The diagnosis is usually established by means of contrast radiology, CT scanning of the abdomen or jejunal biopsy. When systemic spread has occurred a bone marrow examination or liver biopsy may also be helpful.

Treatment of primary intestinal lymphoma depends on the clinical staging of the disease. If limited to one segment, surgical resection (usually with radiotherapy) gives a 50 – 75 per cent five year survival. In the presence of extraintestinal spread the five year survival falls to between 10 and 30 per cent, and in these cases chemotherapy is the treatment of choice. Preliminary surgery or radiotherapy is occasionally used to reduce tumour bulk in patients with extensive disease. In addition to these specific measures, some patients require nutritional support in the form of either enteral or parenteral supplements.

Case 36

Answers

1. Alcoholic Hepatitis.
2. Liver biopsy.
3. Prothrombin time.

Discussion

This patient has alcoholic hepatitis. The clinical presentation of this condition ranges from mild anicteric hepatomegaly to fulminant liver failure. Many cases are misdiagnosed as cholelithiasis because both conditions present with right hypochondrial pain, nausea, jaundice, fever, and leucocytosis. In alcoholic hepatitis the tender liver may also be mistaken for a positive Murphy's sign. To confuse the picture further, gallstones often co-exist. It is vital, to differentiate between the two conditions because inappropriate surgery in alcoholic hepatitis may prove fatal.

To establish the correct diagnosis an accurate assessment of the patient's alcohol intake can be very helpful. Frequently patients are evasive about the quantity drunk and interviewing the spouse or relative can be very informative. The above patient in fact drank half a bottle of vodka on most days and, since fracturing her ribs had been drinking a bottle per day to control pain. Many people with alcoholic hepatitis present after a bout of increased drinking. The diagnosis of cholelithiasis must be questioned if hepatomegaly is present. In alcoholic hepatitis the liver is tender and auscultation may reveal a hepatic bruit. In severe cases, spider naevi, ascites, splenomegaly, and hepatic encephalopathy, may also be present. Although termed alcoholic hepatitis, in 55% of cases the liver function tests show cholestasis. In comparison with extrahepatic cholestasis however the bilirubin tends to be elevated proportionately more than the alkaline phosphatase. The AST tends to be more elevated than the ALT, and it is unusual for either of these to be raised more than 250 IU/ℓ in alcoholic hepatitis. The gamma GT is often grossly elevated, and its disproportionate rise compared with the AST (the AST/gamma GT ratio) suggests alcoholic hepatitis.

Other features that indicate alcohol induced liver disease are reduced albumin, low platelet count and elevated MCV. The low platelets may be secondary to the toxic effect of alcohol on the bone marrow or to hypersplenism. The elevated MCV may arise from the liver disease itself, dietary deficiency of folic acid or haemolysis. The presence of haemolysis and hyperlipidaemia in a patient with alcoholic hepatitis is termed Zieve's Syndrome. Patients with alcoholic hepatitis frequently have a low serum potassium, magnesium and calcium.

To confirm alcoholic hepatitis a liver biopsy should be performed, provided coagulation tests are satisfactory. Although histology will show cholestasis in both alcoholic hepatitis and extrahepatic obstruction, the presence of steatosis (fat deposits in the hepatocytes), marked ballooning of the hepatocytes, and the presence of Mallory's hyaline suggest alcoholic liver disease. If there is any doubt as to the existence of extrahepatic biliary obstruction a CT or ultrasound scan of the liver and biliary tree should be performed, followed by ERCP if necessary.

Other hepatic disorders associated with alcohol excess include fatty liver and cirrhosis. In the former, patients may present with anorexia, nausea, vomiting, weight loss, non-specific abdominal pain, and hepatomegaly. Liver function tests may be normal or show minor increases in the enzymes, but the gamma GT is usually markedly elevated. The MCV is often raised and liver biopsy shows fatty deposits in hepatocytes. The clinical features of alcoholic cirrhosis are similar to other forms of cirrhosis although parotid gland enlargement and Dupuytren's contractures are more common with alcohol abuse.

Abstinence from alcohol is essential in managing these patients. A good diet with adequate calories, protein and vitamins should be given. Liver decompensation and bleeding from oesophageal varices are managed as discussed on pp. 174 and 129. Alcoholic hepatitis is a more severe illness than alcoholic fatty liver. The prothrombin time is the best single predictive factor. The mortality from alcoholic hepatitis is 2% if the prothrombin time is normal, but rises to 33% if prolonged. The presence of Mallory's alcoholic hyaline is also associated with an increased mortality. The long term prognosis of any form of alcoholic liver disease is dependent on whether the patients stop drinking. If they do, and if cirrhosis is not present, the seven-year survival is 80%, but if alcohol intake continues survival is only 40–50%.

110

Case 37

Answers

1. (a) Choledocholithiasis with cholangitis.
   (b) Hepatic abscess.
2. (a) Ultrasound scan
   (b) CT scan
   (c) ERCP or PTC.
3. (a) Cholangitis : Antibiotics + vitamin K
                    Surgical removal of stone *or*
                    ERCP + sphincterotomy
   (b) Hepatic abscess : Antibiotics ± drainage.

Discussion

The two most likely diagnoses in the above patient are choledocholithiasis with cholangitis, and hepatic abscess. Although the patient presents with a pyrexia of uncertain origin there are several clues in the history which point to these diagnoses. The intermittent fever and associated tachycardia, rigors and neutrophil leucocytosis point to an infective disorder and this was confirmed as a gram negative septicaemia on one blood culture. The history of recurrent abdominal discomfort and flatulence together with the raised alkaline phosphatase and gamma GT indicate hepatobiliary disease as the source of this infection. Approximately 15% of patients with cholelithiasis are found to have concomitant choledocholithiasis and the manifestations may range from no symptoms to acute suppurative cholangitis with or without hepatic abscess. Biliary obstruction is accompanied by elevation of the serum alkaline phosphatase and gamma GT and these enzymes may be high in the absence of overt disease and in the presence of a normal or slightly raised bilirubin. The absolute value of the serum bilirubin is a good indication of the degree of obstruction; normal or slightly elevated values suggesting partial obstruction and high values indicating complete or near complete obstruction. Two types of complications may develop from choledocholithiasis: secondary biliary cirrhosis from prolonged obstruction and hepatic abscesses from prolonged or severe cholangitis. Cholangitis almost invariably indicates obstruction to the biliary tree and is caused by bacterial proliferation within the obstructed bile ducts. The clinical manifestations of hepatic abscess are discussed on p. 47. In both of these conditions bacteraemia may be transient with repeated blood cultures negative or intermittently positive.

The liver and biliary tree should initially be studied by means of non-invasive techniques such as ultrasound and CT scanning. Ultrasonography is more widely available than computerized tomography but is of limited value in obese patients and may fail to define the cause of biliary obstruction in the presence of intestinal gas. In the above patient ultrasonography was technically unsatisfactory because of obesity but there was a suggestion of dilated intrahepatic bile ducts. This was confirmed by CT scanning which in addition showed the presence of a dilated common bile duct. Neither investigation defined the nature of the common bile duct obstruction. Although laparotomy could be performed at this stage, a more precise anatomical diagnosis may be provided by either ERCP or percutaneous transhepatic cholangiography (see p. 173). Both of these may define the nature of the obstruction and ERCP may also enable removal of a stone by sphincterotomy or insertion of a stent in the case of malignant obstruction. ERCP confirmed biliary obstruction in this patient and demonstrated the presence of a gall stone in the distal end of the common bile duct.

The treatment of pyogenic liver abscess is discussed on p. 48. Biliary obstruction with cholangitis is usually best treated by urgent surgical drainage of the biliary tree. Pre-operative management should include fluid replacement, antibiotic therapy and correction of any coagulation disturbances caused by vitamin K deficiency. However, in severely ill patients or those with other serious medical disorders the biliary tree may initially be drained by a percutaneous transhepatic approach or by means of ERCP coupled with sphincterotomy. In elderly patients with choledocholithiasis, ERCP with sphincterotomy may be the treatment of choice if local expertise is available, and cholecystectomy may be subsequently performed only if recurrent cholecystitis occurs.

Case 38

Answers

1. (a) Jejunal diverticulosis.
   (b) Barium meal and follow through

2. (a) Folate levels raised in bacterial overgrowth
   (b) (i) Jejunal aspiration
       (ii) ^{14}C xylose breath test.

Discussion

The radiological appearance of multiple fluid levels could represent small bowel obstruction or multiple strictures due to Crohn's disease. The absence of symptoms, however, makes this extremely unlikely. Multiple fluid levels in the absence of obstructive features suggests jejunal diverticulosis, a well recognized cause of bacterial overgrowth, which may be confirmed by barium follow-through examination. Jejunal diverticulosis generally occurs in elderly patients who present with anaemia and steatorrhoea. Multiple diverticula are usually present but occasionally one large diverticulum may be responsible for symptoms. Occult bleeding may occur but frank haemorrhage is rare and ischaemic or traumatic perforation of a diverticulum has been reported. Diarrhoea is usually secondary to steatorrhoea but hydroxylated fatty acids produced by bacterial hydroxylation of malabsorbed fat may also provoke watery diarrhoea. In most patients jejunal diverticulosis is only clinically significant when there is associated bacterial overgrowth.

Malabsorption with a raised serum folate is suggestive of bacterial overgrowth. Under normal circumstances the duodenum is sterile in 82% of subjects, the jejunum in 69%, and the ileum in 55%. Although anaerobic bacteria may be found in small numbers in the ileum they are not usually present in the jejunum. Bacterial overgrowth is present when small bowel aspirates contain more than 10^6 organisms/ml or greater than 10^4 anaerobes/ml. This abnormal proliferation of bacteria, especially anaerobes like Bacteroides, occurs with abnormal gut anatomy (strictures, diverticulosis, internal fistulation, afferent loop, jejuno-ileal bypass etc), abnormal gut motility (pseudo-obstruction, scleroderma, diabetes, etc) and with defective defence mechanisms (hypochlorhydria, immunodeficiency, tropical sprue, etc). Bacterial overgrowth causes malabsorption by a variety of mechanisms. Bacteria deconjugate bile acids causing steatorrhoea, and deaminate dietary proteins and amino acids in the gut lumen resulting in protein malabsorption. Vitamin B_{12} deficiency develops because anaerobes bind B_{12}-intrinsic factor complexes making them unavailable for absorption. Mild mucosal abnormalities occur in jejunal biopsy specimens (inflammatory cell infiltration) and brush border enzyme levels are reduced. Despite malabsorption, serum folate levels are high because some bacteria produce and release folic acid in the gut lumen.

Bacterial overgrowth can be identified in several ways. Culture of jejunal aspirate under anaerobic conditions should yield significant numbers of organisms. Bacterial products, such as organic and fatty acids identified in jejunal juice by chromatography imply the presence of anaerobes. Breath tests are very useful non-invasive tests which provide evidence of bacterial overgrowth. In principle, a substrate is ingested (glycocholic acid, glucose, lactulose, or xylose) which is split by bacterial action releasing a marker substance which can be detected in exhaled air ($^{14}CO_2$ or hydrogen). Unfortunately, unabsorbed substrates passing into the colon will be split by colonic bacteria releasing the marker substances and causing confusion, especially in subjects with fast transit time. ^{14}C glycocholate is split only by anaerobes, which are not always present in bacterial overgrowth, and this substrate gives a 30% false negative rate in some series. As it is principally absorbed in the terminal ileum, ileal malabsorption will cause false positive results. Glucose and lactulose release hydrogen but since this is more difficult to detect in exhaled air than $^{14}CO_2$, larger doses of substrate must be used thus increasing the likelihood of spillover into the colon. ^{14}C labelled xylose as a 1 g dose is normally absorbed high in the small bowel and is split by aerobic bacteria to release $^{14}CO_2$ which can be easily detected. This is probably the most accurate breath test available at present for the detection of bacterial overgrowth. Bacteria degrade tryptophan to indoles which are metabolised by the liver and excreted in the urine as indicans. Increased levels of urinary indicans therefore suggest bacterial overgrowth. Unfortunately, decreased small bowel absorption (e.g. in coeliac disease) allows tryptophan to enter the colon thus producing a false positive result. However, in the absence of severe steatorrhoea urinary indican output over 200 mg/day is a significant result. Serum deconjugated bile acids may also be elevated as a result of increased bacterial deconjugation in the small bowel with subsequent absorption.

The treatment of bacterial overgrowth depends on the causal lesion. Some lesions are amenable to surgical correction (afferent loop, strictures, large solitary diverticulum, blind loop etc) and this is the most appropriate course of action. Most lesions however are not, and treatment consists of supplements of vitamins and nutrients which are easily absorbed (e.g. MCT oils) and eradication of bacteria by antibiotic therapy. Tetracycline and metronidazole are both effective. Neomycin is generally ineffective as it does not kill anaerobes. Treatment may have to be repeated intermittently or continued as long term therapy. Good results have been obtained in patients taking antibiotics for 2 weeks in every month over long periods.

Case 39

Answers

1. Small bowel Crohn's disease.
2. (a) Serial sections of jejunal biopsy to look for granulomata.
   (b) Sigmoidoscopy and biopsy.
3. (a) Reducing the inflammatory process.
   (b) Correction of malnutrition.

Discussion

The history of steatorrhoea, abnormal jejunal biopsy, low serum iron and folate, and abnormal radiology indicate that the jejunum is the major site of his bowel disease. The lack of total villous atrophy on the intestinal biopsy and the presence of an acute inflammatory cell infiltrate rather than a lymphocyte infiltrate make coeliac disease and small bowel lymphoma unlikely. The history of perianal problems and abdominal pain support Crohn's disease as the most likely diagnosis. This could be confirmed by performing serial sections on the jejunal biopsy to look for granulomata or similar search of a rectal biopsy. Twenty-five per cent of patients with Crohn's disease and a normal looking rectal mucosa at endoscopy will exhibit typical non-caseating granulomata on biopsy (*see* p. 190).

Small bowel Crohn's disease can produce profound effects on nutrient absorption. Protein and carbohydrate absorption occur predominantly in the jejunum and therefore proximal disease will lead to nutrient malabsorption as well as calcium, folate, magnesium and iron deficiency, while ileal disease may lead to bile salt and Vitamin B_{12} deficiency. Other factors involved in the development of malnutrition in these patients, include poor intake, active inflammation resulting in increased metabolic needs, and a protein losing enteropathy (*see* p. 126).

The management of upper small bowel Crohn's disease is directed at both reducing the inflammatory response of the condition and correcting accompanying nutritional deficiencies. The patient is initially treated with a high protein diet often supplemented with reconstituted powdered protein extract. Mineral and vitamin replacements are administered if required. Elemental diets using amino acids, peptides, simple carbohydrates and fat are controversial in this condition. Some authorities suggest that such treatment not only improves nutritional status but also reduces activity of the Crohn's disease. However recent evidence suggests that whole protein diets are as well absorbed in these patients and are better tolerated because of their palatability and lower osmotic loads. In severe cases parenteral nutrition, via an indwelling central venous catheter, is required to restore nutritional status.

Therapy to reduce the inflammatory response in proximal small bowel Crohn's differs from that in terminal ileal or colonic forms of the condition. The response to sulphasalazine is poor, possibly related to the fact that substantial sulphasalazine cleavage does not occur at this site (*see* p. 194). It has been suggested, although not proven, that higher doses of 4–6 g/day may be of value in these patients. Prednisolone helps reduce inflammation and may also help correct protein-losing enteropathy. Extensive disease and multiple strictures are a difficult management problem and azathioprine plus corticosteroids may be tried. Some of the symptoms of gastric and duodenal involvement may be improved by H_2 receptor antagonists. Surgery is helpful if there are relatively short areas of involved bowel, isolated strictures, fistulae or abscesses.

Case 40

Answers

1. Acquired hypogammaglobulinaemia with giardiasis.
2. (a) Serum immunoglobulin levels
   (b) Jejunal biopsy
   (c) Microscopy and culture of jejunal juice.
3. (a) Giardiasis
   (b) Associated pernicious anaemia.

Discussion

This patient has acquired hypogammaglobulinaemia and associated *giardia lamblia* infection, producing malabsorption. This diagnosis is suggested by the presence of nodular lymphoid hyperplasia on the barium follow-through; history of chronic sinopulmonary disorders; and blood tests suggesting pernicious anaemia. Nevertheless, other causes of small intestinal malabsorption should be considered. Coeliac disease is less likely since it does not usually cause such severe malabsorption and it is not associated with sinopulmonary disorders. Against a lymphoma is the absence of lymphadenopathy and hepatosplenomegaly. Crohn's disease is unlikely because of the absence of abdominal pain and characteristic abnormalities on the barium meal and follow-through.

The aetiology of acquired hypogammaglobulinaemia is unknown. Patients with this condition have undetectable or low IgA and IgM levels, but normal or only slightly reduced levels of IgG. The initial clinical manifestations are usually recurrent pyogenic infections, particularly sinopulmonary, followed several years later by chronic diarrhoea and malabsorption (50% of cases). Both the diarrhoea and the malabsorption are thought to result from *giardia lamblia* infection or bacterial overgrowth which are present in over 80% of cases. The diagnosis is established by finding characteristic serum immunoglobulin levels and the absence of plasma cells in the lamina propria of jejunal biopsies. The villi are usually normal but some patients have subtotal villous atrophy as in coeliac disease, and may continue to malabsorb after infection has been eradicated. The jejunal biopsy may also show features of nodular lymphoid hyperplasia (*see below*) Jejunal juice should be collected at the time of jejunal biopsy and examined for giardia and excess bacteria. Many other disorders occur with acquired hypogammaglobulinaemia. Nodular lymphoid hyperplasia is found in approximately 60% of cases. This is usually detected on barium studies, as multiple small filling defects in the small intestine, and in jejunal biopsies as lymphoid nodules without plasma cells. A pernicious anaemia-like syndrome occurs in 50% of cases, with achlorhydria, absent intrinsic factor and vitamin B_{12} deficiency. Unlike classical pernicious anaemia autoantibodies are absent and serum gastrin is normal. Gastrointestinal malignancy, especially of the stomach and colon, is more common (15%), particularly in patients with nodular lymphoid hyperplasia. A rare complication is ulcerative jejuno-ileitis producing severe diarrhoea and malabsorption and this is often fatal. Other reported associations include Crohn's disease, ulcerative colitis, pancreatic insufficiency, cholelithiasis, liver disease, and other autoimmune diseases.

An essential component of treatment is eradication of small bowel infection, using metronidazole for giardiasis and either metronidazole or tetracycline for bacterial overgrowth. It is often necessary to give prolonged treatment for 3–6 weeks. Gluten free diets, replacement immunoglobulins, or fresh frozen plasma infusions are of little benefit but are worth trying if malabsorption or recurrent infection persist and especially if there is subtotal villous atrophy. Steroids are of no benefit and may exacerbate infection.

There are many other types of primary immune-deficiency disorders affecting the small bowel (*See Table 5*), the commonest being selective IgA Deficiency (which occurs in about 1 in 500 people). Many patients are asymptomatic since normal IgM compensates for the absent IgA. Symptomatic cases present with chronic sinopulmonary disorders, diarrhoea and malabsorption. It is also important to distinguish primary from secondary hypoglobulinaemia, which can occur in protein losing enteropathy (*see* p. 66).

Table 5: Primary immune-deficiency disorders affecting the small bowel

Immunodeficiency	*Gastrointestinal features*
Antibody (B-cell) defects	
X-linked congenital hypogammaglobulinaemia.	Malabsorption and diarrhoea
Acquired hypogammaglobulinaemia (Common variable or late onset)	Giardiasis and bacterial overgrowth; nodular lymphoid hyperplasia; pernicious anaemia; proctocolitis; malignancy
Selective IgA deficiency	Pernicious anaemia; coeliac disease; Crohn's disease
Selective IgM deficiency	Ulcerative colitis; Crohn's disease; Whipple's disease
Selective IgD deficiency	Coeliac disease
T-cell defects	
Congenital thymic aplasia (Di–George Syndrome)	Malabsorption and diarrhoea
Combined B and T-cell defects	
Combined immunodeficiency disease	Malabsorption and diarrhoea
Immunodeficiency with ataxia, telangiectasia	Vitamin B_{12} malabsorption; gastric carcinoma
Cellular immunodeficiency with abnormal immunoglobulin synthesis (Nezelof's Syndrome)	Malabsorption and candidiasis
Immunodeficiency with eczema, thrombocytopaenia (Wiskott–Aldrich Syndrome)	Malabsorption and bloody diarrhoea

Case 41

Answers

1. (a) Diabetic ketoacidosis
   (b) Emphysematous cholecystitis.
2. None.
3. (a) Fluid replacement
   (b) Insulin
   (c) Antibiotics.

Discussion

The patient had diabetic ketoacidosis and acute emphysematous cholecystitis. The history and physical signs, together with the results of investigations, are typical of acute cholecystitis and the severity of toxaemia with the presence of gas in the vicinity of the gall bladder highly suggestive of emphysematous cholecystitis. There is a higher incidence of cholesterol gallstones in diabetics compared with the general population and 20% of all patients with emphysematous cholecystitis have diabetes mellitus.

Emphysematous cholecystitis is a form of acute cholecystitis in which the gall bladder and occasionally the bile ducts and pericholecystic area contain gas. It is caused by infection with gas-producing bacteria, in particular *Clostridium welchii, Escherichia coli* and anaerobic streptococci. Clinically, the disorder resembles the usual type of acute cholecystitis but men outnumber women by 3 to 1 and patients have more severe pain and toxaemia. A substantial number of these patients have no gallstones and it has been suggested that the disorder is due to sudden interruption of the blood supply to the gall bladder. Plain abdominal X-ray is often diagnostic showing gas in the lumen and wall of the gall bladder. Further investigations that may help establish the diagnosis include repeated blood cultures and CT scanning of the right hypochondrium. In the above patient the clinical picture and X-ray appearance was adequate to make a definite diagnosis.

The three main priorities in managing this patient are fluid replacement, administration of insulin and appropriate parenteral antibiotics. The diabetic ketoacidosis should respond to adequate fluid and electrolyte replacement plus parenteral insulin. If no organism is cultured from blood cultures, a combination of an aminoglycoside and metronidazole, given intravenously, should cover the range of responsible organisms. Once the patient is stable, laparotomy and cholecystectomy should be performed, although in some seriously ill patients a cholecystotomy may be preferable as an initial procedure. The morbidity and mortality of emphysematous cholecystitis is substantially higher than for uncomplicated acute cholecystitis. Gas gangrene of the abdominal wall is a rare outcome. The above patient responded well to therapy and a cholecystectomy was subsequently performed.

Case 42

Answers

1. Travellers' diarrhoea.
2. (a) Avoidance of contaminated food
   (b) Prophylactic antibiotics
   (c) Bismuth subsalicylate.
3. (a) Oral rehydration
   (b) Early refeeding
   (c) Co-trimoxazole.

Discussion

Several diagnoses need to be considered in this patient. An acute exacerbation of his inflammatory bowel disease could explain many features of his illness but the absence of blood in the stool and the sigmoidoscopic appearances make colitis unlikely. It is most likely that this patient has developed an attack of traveller's diarrhoea. His recent arrival in an endemic area and the sudden onset of watery diarrhoea with fever and abdominal cramps are typical features. Patients with pre-existing bowel disease may be more prone to develop severe diarrhoea when exposed to enteric infections.

Many infective agents can cause travellers' diarrhoea but 70% of attacks are due to toxin-producing *Escherichia coli* organisms. Ingested organisms produce a heat-stable toxin, a heat-labile toxin, or both, and these stimulate active intestinal secretion of water and electrolytes. *Giardia lamblia, campylobacter, salmonella* and *shigella* are less frequent causes of travellers' diarrhoea and *cholera* is even more unusual.

As transmission of travellers' diarrhoea is usually via contaminated food or water the risks of developing diarrhoea are considerably reduced if uncooked food and untreated water (or ice) are avoided. Vaccination against toxigenic *E. coli* is not available at present since a single strain may produce more than one toxin. Various antibiotics (e.g. doxycycline and co-trimoxazole) have been shown to be effective in preventing travellers' diarrhoea. Despite its effectiveness, antibiotic prophylaxis is not recommended for routine travel for several reasons. Antibiotic resistant strains of enterotoxigenic *E. coli* are already common in some areas and as the genes for toxin production may be linked to those for antibiotic resistance, these drugs would favour the emergence of resistant toxin-producing coliforms. It is also possible that antibiotic prophylaxis could predispose travellers to more serious infections as the inoculum of *salmonellae* needed to cause infection is less when normal gut flora is suppressed by antibiotics. If prophylactic treatment is discontinued whilst in a high risk area the likelihood of developing diarrhoea is even greater. Adverse drug effects are also a potential problem. Antibiotic prophylaxis may be indicated in certain individuals, e.g. travellers with serious underlying conditions in whom diarrhoea would present difficult management problems, serving members of the armed forces and people on important short stay business trips. Bismuth subsalicylate 60 ml 6 hourly taken throughout the visit can reduce the incidence of travellers' diarrhoea but the large volumes of medicine required make it an inconvenient form of prophylaxis.

The diagnosis of travellers' diarrhoea is often made clinically and the self-limiting diarrhoea has usually ceased by the time the results of stool culture are available. Fortunately all acute secretory diarrhoeas can be treated using similar general principles. Persistent diarrhoea (longer than 3 days) or stools containing blood or mucus suggest the need for further investigation. The treatment of traveller's diarrhoea depends on its severity, the major clinical problems being dehydration and acidosis due to faecal fluid and electrolyte losses. Shocked patients, or those too weak to drink, require intravenous fluids but traveller's diarrhoea rarely causes such severe dehydration. Most patients can be rehydrated with oral solutions containing Na^+, K^+ and HCO_3^- to replete electrolyte losses and glucose to stimulate absorption. Sodium chloride coupled absorption is inhibited by *E. coli* toxin but glucose linked Na^+

absorption is unaffected, even in the presence of marked intestinal secretion. Oral rehydration therapy is not designed to stop diarrhoea, merely to replace losses until the diarrhoea ceases. Several proprietary formulations are available but their composition is not ideal and the solution developed by the World Health Organisation is therefore recommended. Vomiting is usually due to fluid depletion and acidosis and rarely causes oral therapy to fail. Early re-feeding, as soon as appetite permits, will help to maintain weight, and restore well-being more rapidly. Drug therapy in mild attacks of travellers' diarrhoea is aimed at symptomatic relief. A 5 day course of co-trimoxazole reduces diarrhoea and shortens attacks and is valuable therapy in severe attacks. Our patient was treated with oral rehydration solution, early refeeding and co-trimoxazole and made a rapid recovery.

Case 43

Answers

1. (a) Crohn's disease.
   (b) Tuberculosis.
   (c) Rectal cancer with spread.
2. (a) Sigmoidoscopy with rectal biopsy,
   (b) Chest X-ray.
3. Excludes chronic fissure-in-ano.

Discussion

The combination of fleshy anal tags, sinuses and a painless anal fissure all suggest perianal Crohn's disease. The other differential diagnoses to consider include extensive carcinoma of the rectum, tuberculosis, syphilis and lympho-granuloma inguinale. A rectal biopsy is vital to distinguish between the above and sigmoidoscopy, colonoscopy and barium follow-through examination of the small intestine may be required to delineate the extent of the disease. A chest X-ray is required to eliminate pulmonary tuberculosis.

The incidence of perianal manifestations in patients with Crohn's disease varies between 40 and 90% depending on the diagnostic criteria selected. Associated lesions in the large bowel are seen more frequently than small bowel disease. The perianal problems may precede bowel involvement by some years and thus careful follow up is required. A variety of lesions are encountered in the perianal region but, with the exception of abscesses, most are pain less. Skin tags are oedematous folds of perianal skin and can occur with any cause of pruritis ani. True haemorrhoids are probably rare in Crohn's disease, the majority of haemorrhoid-like lesions being skin tags. Multiple fissures are characteristic of this condition and in contrast to the usual fissure-in-ano, are painless and sited laterally Anal stenosis is a sequel to long standing fissures and ulcers, but despite producing a tiny lumen rarely seems to cause symptoms Fistulae tend to be symptomatic only when the track become blocked and an abscess develops or when there is a large connec tion with the vagina or bladder.

The typical patient is over 50 years and has symptoms of diar rhoea accompanied by mucus and blood. Many have co-existing diverticular disease and this should not be accepted as the cause o their bowel symptoms. A less well recognized symptom is faeca incontinence which patients find particularly distressing and embarrassing to discuss. Rectal pressure studies show reduction o the resting and maximum squeeze pressure of the anal sphincter i perianal Crohn's disease, and a major problem is inability to retain fluid load. Most patients with severe perianal disease have a combi nation of poor anal sphincter tone, reduced rectal capacity and sinuses or fistulae, resulting in incontinence. The general appear ance of perianal Crohn's is very striking, but unless there is inconti nence or infection, symptoms may be relatively slight.

Perianal lesions often improve after active disease elsewhere ha been treated. There is no evidence that specific therapy wit corticosteroids or sulphasalazine is of value. Azathioprine an metronidazole have been shown to help some patients in controlle trials. The risks of immunosuppression, however do not justify th use of azathioprine except in the most disabling cases. Metronidazol by reducing bacterial infection may allow normal healing to tak place and should be tried in symptomatic patients. Many requir this drug for up to 9 months before achieving benefit and unfortu nately most will relapse when the drug is withdrawn (see p. 194).

Surgery is only required for drainage of abscesses and should b as limited as possible. Extensive local surgery can produce incont nence and fistula formation and should therefore be avoided. Ana strictures require gentle dilatation when there is difficulty in defaecation. If there are major problems from fistulae to the vagina or bladder then surgery is needed with total excision of the rectum. This will result in healing of most perianal lesions and the recurrence rate in proximal bowel is low. The overall prognosis in uncomplicated perianal Crohn's disease is good, despite the rather florid appearance.

Case 44

Answers

1. (a) Erythromycin induced liver damage
   (b) Extrahepatic obstruction
   (c) Viral hepatitis.
2. (a) Abdominal ultrasound scan.
   (b) Serology for viral hepatitis.
   (c) Liver biopsy.

Discussion

This nurse had erythromycin induced liver damage. In view of the clinical and biochemical features of cholestasis exclusion of extrahepatic obstruction is essential. The prodromal symptoms would be compatible with viral hepatitis but the LFT's are not typical. The finding of atypical lymphocytes suggest the possibility of infectious mononucleosis, although this is less likely in the absence of lymphadenopathy.

The possibility of drug induced liver damage should always be considered whenever there is hepatic dysfunction. The patient should be questioned as to what drugs have been taken; when taken; how long for; and whether they have been taken in the past. A check of the general practitioner's records, hospital case notes, drug charts, and anaesthetic records, may be of value. The periods during which drugs were taken should then be plotted against the time course of the illness to establish any relationship. Associated features of an immunological reaction, such as fever, rash, or eosinophilia, should be sought and other causes of hepato-biliary dysfunction excluded. Pre-existing chronic liver disease may be identified by clinical examination and review of any previous liver function tests. Acute disorders such as a viral hepatitis or extra-hepatic obstruction should be excluded by testing for the hepatitis B surface antigen and the hepatitis A IgM antibody, as well as Paul–Bunnell test and an abdominal ultrasound scan. Usually, no further investigations are needed and the effect of stopping the implicated drug(s) is observed. Liver biopsy is reserved for patients with suspected pre-existing liver disease or those who fail to respond to withdrawal of the drug(s). Rechallenge with the drug should not be performed since there is a risk of inducing fulminant hepatic failure.

Erythromycin induced liver damage is most commonly associated with the estolate ester but has been reported with the proprionate and ethyl succinate esters. Clinical features develop 1 – 4 weeks after starting therapy, but may occur earlier if there has been previous exposure to the drug. Ninety per cent of patients develop jaundice, and 75% have a prodromal phase, lasting approximately 2 days with fatigue, malaise, anorexia, nausea or vomiting. Pruritis, right upper quadrant pain, and intermittent fever occur in 40% of cases. About 30% develop hepatomegaly, and 15% lymphadenopathy. The blood count may show eosinophilia or atypical lymphocytes and the liver function tests usually show a cholestatic pattern. Liver biopsy in erythromycin induced damage shows centrilobular cholestasis but no bile lakes or inter lobular bile duct cholestasis which are found in extrahepatic obstruction. There may be some hepatocellular injury manifested by ballooning of the

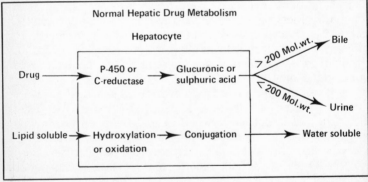

Figure 2 Stages involved in the hepatic metabolism of a lipid soluble drug. Following intrahepatic hydroxylation or oxidation and conjugation the drug is excreted into bile or urine depending on its molecular weight

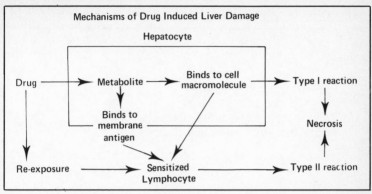

Figure 3 Possible mechanisms of type I and type II hepatotoxic drug reactions

hepatocytes and the presence of acidophil bodies, but these changes are normally less marked than in viral hepatitis.

The liver enzymes convert lipid soluble drugs into water soluble metabolites which are excreted in the urine or bile (*see Figure 2*). It has been suggested that drug induced liver cell damage results from either toxic metabolites (type I) or an immunological reaction (type II, *Figure 3*). The former reaction is normally prevented by intracellular glutathione, which preferentially combines with toxic metabolites thus preventing cell damage. If the stores of glutathione become depleted, as in paracetamol overdose, cell necrosis occurs. However, not all drug reactions fit into one or other group, and some of type II reactions may be caused by a genetic susceptibility, toxicity being biochemically mediated.

Table 6: Drug induced liver cell damage resulting from toxic metabolites (Type I) or immunological reaction (Type II)

Type I reactions	Type II reactions
Paracetamol overdose	Halothane
Tetracycline	Methyldopa
Methotrexate	Isoniazid
Azathioprine	Rifampicin
6-Mercaptopurine	Erythromycin
Cyclophosphamide	Sulphonamides
Carbon tetrachloride	Nitrofurantoin
(dry cleaning agents,	Perhexilene
fire extinguishers)	Phenothiazines
	Imipramine

Case 45

Answers

1. (a) Protein losing enteropathy.
   (b) Radio-labelled albumin study.
2. (a) Primary intestinal lymphangiectasia.
   (b) Jejunal biopsy or lymphangiography.
3. Low fat diet.

Discussion

The low albumin and decreased concentration of all three immunoglobulins, in the presence of normal renal function, are highly suggestive of a protein-losing gastroenteropathy. Dietary intake of protein was adequate and renal protein loss insignificant. Apart from a raised alkaline phosphatase due to bone growth, liver function tests were normal and lowering of all three immunoglobulins is not a feature of hepatic cirrhosis. The most likely cause of this patient's low serum protein is therefore loss from the gastrointestinal tract.

Hypoproteinaemia with enteric loss of plasma protein was first described in 1957. The gastrointestinal tract plays a small but significant role in the normal metabolism and degradation of serum proteins, and studies using radio-labelled albumin suggest that it accounts for approximately 10% of normal turnover. In disorders associated with inflammation or ulceration of the intestinal mucosa, dilatation of the lymphatic channels or alteration in intestinal permeability, excessive protein loss may occur (*see Table 7*). In addition to albumin and gamma globulins, a number of other plasma proteins are lost including fibrinogen, lipoproteins, transferrin and caeruloplasmin. However, the main manifestation of such loss is dependent oedema, resulting from lowered plasma osmotic pressure and secondary hyperaldosteronism. Hypogammaglobulinaemia rarely predisposes to infection.

The most likely pathological diagnosis in the above patient is primary or idiopathic intestinal lymphangiectasia. This condition usually affects children or young adults and is characterized by asymmetrical peripheral oedema, hypoproteinaemia, lymphocytopenia and mild gastrointestinal symptoms, with or without steatorrhoea. In the above case asymmetry of the oedema and

Table 7: Causes of enteric loss of plasma proteins

Mucosal ulceration	Gastric carcinoma or lymphoma
	Multiple gastric ulcers
	Crohn's disease
	Colonic cancer
Mucosal disease without ulceration	Menetrier's disease
	Coeliac disease
	Tropical sprue
	Whipple's disease
Lymphatic abnormalities	Primary lymphangiectasia
	Lymphoma
	Constrictive pericarditis
	Parasitic infestation
	Tuberculosis

lymphopenia are important clues to this diagnosis. The lack of response to a strict gluten free diet makes coeliac disease less likely and the other disorders listed in the table are uncommon in this age group. The mean age of onset of idiopathic lymphangiectasia is 10 years and most reported cases develop symptoms before the age of 30 years. The pathogenesis of the increased protein and lymphocyte loss is thought to be related to increased lymphatic pressure leading to rupture and discharge of the lymphatic contents into the gut lumen. The cause of the increased lymphatic pressure in patients with primary lymphangiectasia has not been identified.

Enteric protein loss may be confirmed by giving an intravenous injection of radio-labelled albumin and collecting stools for at least 4 days. Normal subjects excrete less than 1% of this labelled albumin while in protein losing enteropathy over 2% is lost. This is however a cumbersome technique and there is evidence that measurement of the faecal clearance of alpha-1 antitrypsin may provide similar information. The two best techniques for diagnosing intestinal lymphangiectasia are lymphangiography and peroral jejunal biopsy. Lymphangiography shows evidence of peripheral and visceral lymphatic hypoplasia in primary lymphangiectasia and jejunal biopsy will show dilatation of the intramucosal lymphatics with distortion of the villous architecture. Occasionally this condition is patchy in distribution and multiple jejunal biopsies may be necessary. Jejunal biopsy per se cannot distinguish between primary and secondary forms of lymphangiectasia and if there is any doubt as to the cause, lymphangiography and barium examination should be performed.

A low fat diet supplemented, if necessary, with medium chain triglycerides reduces lymphatic flow and produces clinical remission in most patients. The prognosis in patients with primary lymphangiectasia is very good. In those who fail to respond, lymphangiography may define a segment of bowel with severe involvement that may be amenable to surgical resection.

Case 46

Answers

1. Gaucher's disease;
2. Autosomal recessive inheritance.
3. (a) Vasopressin infusion.
   (b) Balloon tamponade.
   (c) Injection sclerotherapy.

Discussion

Bilateral hip disease with flattening of the femoral heads in a young man with portal hypertension suggests the possibility of Gaucher's disease and splenectomy in childhood is consistent with this diagnosis. The family history may be helpful but since Gaucher's disease is inherited as an autosomal recessive condition family history of the disease may be absent.

The commonest form of Gaucher's disease is characterized by gross splenic enlargement and hepatomegaly due to accumulation of glucosylceramide resulting from deficiency of the enzyme, glucosylceramide β glucosidase. Painful expanding deposits occur in bone and can cause softening of the femoral heads. The enlarged spleen results in thrombocytopenia, necessitating splenectomy in some cases. Liver function tests are only mildly abnormal but portal hypertension may develop. Recurrent pulmonary infections, skin pigmentation and pingueculae also occur. Acid phosphatase, not inhibited by L-tartrate and therefore easily distinguished from prostatic acid phosphatase, is markedly increased. Examination of bone marrow or splenic aspirates may reveal typical Gaucher's cells. Enzyme replacement therapy is so far experimental, and no specific treatment is available at present.

Patients with bleeding varices should be screened for coagulation defects and appropriate corrective action taken. Blood transfusion is essential and attempts should be made to stop the bleeding. Continuous infusion of vasopressin (0.4 u/min) is more effective than bolus doses in arresting variceal haemorrhage but if bleeding persists, balloon tamponade with a properly placed Sengstaken–Blakemore tube will invariably stop haemorrhage from lower oesophageal varices. A four lumen tube should always be used allowing aspiration of the upper oesophagus and thus preventing inhalation of blood. Unfortunately rebleeding after deflating the balloon is common (60% of cases). Injection of sclerosant into or around the varices before or after control of haemorrhage by balloon tamponade, is successful in the initial control of bleeding in 96% of cases. Results are equally good using fibreoptic endoscopes and the rigid oesophagoscope. Transhepatic embolization of varices is often effective (80% of cases) in stopping acute bleeding but the technique requires considerable expertise. If bleeding cannot be controlled by these measures emergency transection of the oesophagus, devascularization operations or stapling gun transection may be effective although operative mortality is appreciable. Emergency porta-caval shunt has a mortality of 50% and is not recommended for the initial control of active bleeding.

After control of haemorrhage, steps should be taken to prevent rebleeding. Long term beta blocker therapy sufficient to slow the resting pulse rate by 25%, may reduce portal pressure and in selected patients prevent rebleeding. Repeated courses of variceal sclerotherapy reduce the risk of rebleeding by obliterating varices and the low morbidity of this procedure makes it an attractive option, especially in patients who are unsuitable for major surgery. Oesophageal transection is frequently followed by rebleeding and is therefore unsuitable for long term control of bleeding. Elective shunt surgery in properly selected patients may still be of value. Child's classification into groups A, B and C taking into account serum bilirubin, albumin, nutritional state and the presence of ascites or encephalopathy is useful as it correlates well with operative mortality and survival during the first post-operative year (Pugh's modification is similar but uses prothrombin time instead of nutritional state). Child's C patients are not suitable for shunting while those in group A are ideal candidates. Patients in group B may be difficult to assess and each individual should be reviewed jointly by surgeon and physician. Portacaval shunts are followed by encephalopathy in 20–40% of patients whilst selective shunts (e.g. distal splenorenal) cause encephalopathy in 5–20%. Although rebleeding after shunt surgery occurs in <5% of patients, the natural history of liver disease is not altered and overall survival is approximately 50% at 5 years. Shunt surgery is particularly useful however, for extrahepatic portal vein occlusion and hepatic vein obstruction (Budd–Chiari Syndrome). The best option for the prevention of rebleeding from oesophageal varices will therefore depend on the state of the patient, local availability of techniques and the underlying disease process.

Case 47

Answers

1. Polyarteritis nodosa.
2. Corticosteroids.
3. (a) Malnutrition due to short bowel syndrome:
   (b) Treatment with enteral and parenteral nutrition.

Discussion

The combination of small bowel infarction, asthma, supraventricular arrythmia, raised ESR, eosinophilia and proteinuria suggests polyarteritis nodosa. This is a necrotising arteritis of unknown aetiology affecting mainly medium and small arteries. Twenty-five per cent of patients have a positive Hepatitis B antigen but the significance of this is unclear and the pathogenesis is probably related to immune complex deposition in blood vessels, provoking a vasculitis. Other symptoms include malaise, weight loss, myalgia, arthralgia, skin rashes and mononeuritis multiplex. Gastrointestinal involvement is frequent, with 50–70% of patients having abdominal symptoms. Abdominal pain occurs in 15–40%, characteristically in the right upper quadrant and epigastrium, and may simulate peptic ulcer, appendicitis or cholecystitis. Up to 45% of patients have anorexia, nausea, vomiting and diarrhoea, or constipation. Around 20% develop gastrointestinal haemorrhage which may arise from shallow ischaemic ulcers anywhere in the gut, the small bowel being the commonest site. Approximately 5% of patients may develop small bowel infarction. Intestinal obstruction, perforation and intussusception have also been described.

The diagnosis of polyarteritis nodosa is often difficult to establish. Selective coeliac axis and renal angiography are thought to be the most accurate investigations. Muscle biopsy is less helpful and is positive in only 35% of cases.

The mainstay of therapy is high dose corticosteroids (40–60 mg prednisolone) which induces a remission in the majority of patients. Cyclophosphamide (3 mg/kg/day) may be added to steroid therapy in resistant cases and in the severely affected, plasmaphaeresis should be considered. Laparotomy should not be delayed if small bowel infarction is suspected. If a remission is induced, the corticosteroid or cyclophosphamide dosage is maintained at the lowest level that will suppress manifestations of the disorder. Renal involvement is the usual cause of death and hypertension occurs at some stage in most patients. Providing the patient survives the first few weeks, 5 year survival is around 50–60%.

The histology of the resected specimen from our patient showed moderate vasculitis of arterioles. She was treated with corticosteroids and made a good recovery with complete remission of disease activity. The major problem was maintaining her nutritional status after such extensive small bowel resection. A normal diet resulted in marked diarrhoea and steatorrhoea associated with weight loss. Enteral feeding was also unsuccessful and she is now maintained on long term home parenteral nutrition, 4–5 days per week, eating food the rest of the time.

Case 48

Answers

1. (a) Ulcerative colitis is most likely.
   (b) Crohn's colitis.
   (c) Pseudomembranous colitis.
   (d) Enteric infection.

2. (a) Stool microscopy and culture.
   (b) Repeat abdominal X-ray.
   (c) Sigmoidoscopy with biopsy.
3. (a) Continuing bloody diarrhoea.
   (b) Persisting pyrexia.
   (c) Tachycardia.

Discussion

The differential diagnosis in this age group is ulcerative colitis, Crohn's colitis, pseudomembranous colitis, and enteric infections, such as Campylobacter enteritis or bacillary dysentery. Although 50% of patients with Crohn's colitis do have rectal bleeding, it is usually not marked. The narrow anal sphincter might favour Crohn's disease, but there were no other features of perianal Crohn's (*see* p. 121). Pseudomembranous colitis is a possibility in view of the recent antibiotic therapy, but the 4 year history of intermittent blood stained diarrhoea makes this, as well as other infective disorders, unlikely. Nevertheless, patients with inflammatory bowel disease may develop enteric infections and these may mimic or precipitate an acute relapse of the disease.

This patient had features of severe ulcerative colitis in that she had blood stained diarrhoea more than 6 times per day, pyrexia, tachycardia, anaemia, and hypoalbuminaemia. Investigation of these severely ill patients must be limited because barium enema and colonoscopy may either precipitate toxic dilatation or cause perforation. Diagnosis therefore rests on repeated stool microscopy and culture to exclude infective diarrhoea, repeat abdominal X-rays, and sigmoidoscopy. The plain abdominal X-ray may be helpful in diagnosing ulcerative colitis, as loss of haustrations and a feathery ulcerated margin may be seen in the gas filled colon, and would also exclude toxic dilatation. The extent of colonic involvement can sometimes be estimated from the presence of faeces proximal to the gas filled ulcerated bowel ('proximal constipation'). Careful sigmoidoscopy, without excess air insufflation, is safe and helpful. In this patient the rectal mucosa was granular, hyperaemic, friable and haemorrhagic with loss of the blood vessel pattern. There were no ulcers with overlying membranes to suggest pseudomembranous colitis and microbiological studies of the stools were negative.

The management of a severe attack of acute ulcerative colitis consists of correcting fluid and electrolyte imbalance and anaemia, giving high dose intravenous steroids (hydrocortisone 100 mg up to 4 times per day) and improving nutritional status. In severe attacks the latter is best done by parenteral feeding. With less severe attacks, enteric feeding using a liquid or low residue diet may be possible. Anti-diarrhoeal drugs must be used with caution, particularly opiate derivatives, as they may precipitate toxic dilatation. It is vital to monitor temperature, pulse, stool frequency and appearance, and abdominal girth which, in conjunction with repeated abdominal X-rays, is important in the detection of toxic dilatation. Continuing pyrexia, tachycardia, bloody diarrhoea, increasing abdominal girth, radiological dilatation of the colon, and falling haemoglobin and albumin, are important indicators for surgical intervention. The aim is to operate early before toxic dilatation and perforation develop, since these are associated with a mortality of 40–50%. Depending on the severity of the acute attack and the response to medical treatment, surgical intervention should be contemplated within 2–5 days. If toxic dilatation is present on admission, surgery should be undertaken immediately after resuscitation. The above patient failed to improve on medical treatment and total colectomy, with preservation of the rectal stump was performed.

Systemic complications are numerous. The skin lesions include erythema nodosum (2%) and pyoderma gangrenosum, usually sited on the shins. Ten percent of patients develop arthritis and 3% sacroiliitis or ankylosing spondylitis. These arthritic and skin lesions are often accompanied by conjunctivitis, iritis, or episcleritis. About 6% of patients develop aphthous ulceration of the mouth during the acute attack. Thromboembolism is more likely in severe attacks (5%) due to thrombocytosis, increased fibrinogen and coagulation factors, hypovolaemia and immobility. Hepatobiliary disease occurs in 2% of patients (fatty change, pericholangitis, sclerosing cholangitis, chronic active hepatitis, cirrhosis and cholangiocarcinoma).

Case 49

Answers

1. Vagotomy and cholecystectomy.
2. Dumping syndrome (*see* p. 164).
3. (a) Barium meal and follow-through.
   (b) Jejunal biopsy.
   (c) Thyroid function tests.

Discussion

Troublesome diarrhoea occurs in approximately 10% of patients after truncal vagotomy and this may be severe in up to 1%. Two syndromes of diarrhoea have been described: a continuous form characterized by 3 or more watery stools per day and an episodic form with attacks of explosive diarrhoea and incontinence alternating with normal bowel action. Faecal excretion of bile salts is increased after truncal vagotomy and the incidence of diarrhoea is significantly increased in those patients who have had cholecystectomy. Thus in the above patient, the two surgical procedures, truncal vagotomy and cholecystectomy, are primarily responsible for the development of diarrhoea and mild steatorrhoea.

Several factors have been implicated in the pathogenesis of post-vagotomy diarrhoea and steatorrhoea. Truncal vagotomy increases emptying of liquids, diminishes pancreatic enzyme response to eating, may reduce duodenal bile salt concentration and accelerates the transit of chyme through the small intestine. Faecal bile salt output is increased in patients with post-vagotomy diarrhoea and abnormal delivery of bile salts into the colon may induce the diarrhoea. There is no evidence that alteration in small intestinal bacteria, epithelial morphology or mucosal ion fluxes contribute to the diarrhoea and mild steatorrhoea. Occasionally, vagotomy may unmask latent coeliac disease or lactose intolerance by increasing the concentration of nutrients in the proximal small bowel (see p. 165). Faecal incontinence develops when the anal sphincter is incompetent or the capacity of the normal sphincter mechanism is overwhelmed by large volume watery diarrhoea. Anorectal surgery is an important cause of abnormal anal sphincter function but similar abnormalities may result from a pudendal nerve neuropathy following obstetric procedures such as forceps delivery. The development of diarrhoea in patients with abnormal anal sphincter function may thus precipitate or exacerbate incontinence.

Post-vagotomy diarrhoea occurs commonly in the early postoperative period and usually subsides spontaneously. If it persists after 6 weeks however, further investigations are indicated. In the above patient, thyrotoxicosis should be excluded and a jejunal biopsy obtained to exclude coeliac disease and hypolactasia; both of which may be exacerbated by gastric surgery (see p. 165). A barium meal and follow-through is occasionally helpful if it shows rapid gastric emptying and intestinal transit.

Post-vagotomy diarrhoea usually responds to antidiarrhoeal agents such as loperamide and codeine phosphate. In refractory cases or those in whom a cholecystectomy has also been performed a trial of the bile salt binding agent, cholestyramine, is indicated. Patients with steatorrhoea usually benefit from a reduction in fat intake. If diarrhoea is severe and unresponsive to these measures further surgery, such as pyloric reconstruction or jejunal interposition, may be warranted.

Case 50

Answers

1. Obstructive jaundice due to malignant carcinoid tumour.
2. (a) Urine 5 HIAA.
   (b) Flush provocation tests.
3. (a) Arterial embolisation of liver metastases.
   (b) Cytotoxic Chemotherapy.
   (c) 5HT antagonists and bradykinin inhibitors.
   (d) Surgery.

Discussion

The differential diagnosis of a bile duct stricture at the porta hepatis must include cholangiocarcinoma and pressure from enlarged (usually malignant) lymph nodes at the porta hepatis. A localized indentation presumably due to lymphadenopathy occasionally occurs in primary biliary cirrhosis but this is never associated with dilated intrahepatic ducts. Benign post-operative strictures rarely occur at the porta hepatis and this patient gave no history of biliary surgery. The patient has several manifestations of the carcinoid syndrome suggesting that metastatic spread from a carcinoid tumour to nodes at the porta hepatis was responsible for the jaundice and biochemical findings.

Carcinoid tumour accounts for only 0.5–1% of all gastrointestinal tumours and is classed histologically as an argentaffinoma. The

commonest site is the appendix but these tumours rarely metastasise. Ileal tumours are often small and multiple but metastasise
more frequently. Primary carcinoid tumours occur less commonly in
other parts of the gastrointestinal tract, bronchus and ovary. The
classical carcinoid syndrome only occurs when tumour products
enter directly into the systemic circulation either from liver
secondaries or from primary tumours not drained by the portal
venous system (e.g. stomach, bronchus, ovary). Almost all patients
complain of flushing and over 80% have diarrhoea, although the
stools can vary in the same patient from almost normal to watery.
Flushing may be precipitated by certain foods (cheese, salt, alcohol,
etc) and usually affects the face and/or the neck. Paroxysms
normally last a few minutes but bronchial carcinoids may cause prolonged flushing over several days and facial oedema. A variety of
skin lesions occur with the carcinoid syndrome including facial
telangiectasia, red/blue discolouration of the face and a pellagra-
like rash. Asthma occurs in 20% of cases and hyperventilation or
bronchoconstriction may occur during flushing. Even small tumours
can produce an intense fibrotic reaction resulting in intestinal
obstruction, retroperitoneal fibrosis or constrictive pericarditis,
depending on the site of the tumour and its deposits. Valvular heart
lesions occur including pulmonary stenosis and tricuspid incompe-
tence and these may precipitate congestive cardiac failure.

The diagnosis may be confirmed by demonstrating increased
urinary excretion of hydroxyindoles, which are metabolites of
5 hydroxytryptamine (5HT) produced by the tumour. Blood levels of
5HT are more sensitive but difficult to measure. Carcinoid tumours
also produce a variety of other vasoactive substances including
bradykinins and histamine, which may mediate the flushing. Flush
provocation may occasionally be helpful; 10 ml of ethanol orally
causes flushing in 30% of cases and 5 μg of adrenaline IV, in almost
all. These provocation tests also increase urinary hydroxyindole
excretion. Histological confirmation of the diagnosis is important as
carcinoid tumours are amenable to therapy. The demonstration and
subsequent biopsy of liver metastases is frequently successful in
providing a definitive diagnosis but laparotomy may be necessary
in some cases. Extraintestinal carcinoids will be diagnosed by
appropriate tests (e.g. chest X-ray, pelvic examination etc).

Since the occurrence of carcinoid syndrome usually indicates the
presence of liver metastases, treatment is palliative. Fortunately
these tumours are slow growing and chemotherapy together with a
reduction in tumour mass may be effective. Methysergide, Ketanse-
rin (5HT antagonists) and alpha adrenergic blockers are useful

symptomatic treatments for the diarrhoea, while phenothiazines (bradykinin inhibitors) may help control the flushing. Arterial embolization of the liver, causing necrosis of secondary deposits may be useful in some cases. However, in many centres, reduction of tumour mass may only be achieved by hepatic resection. The most effective cytotoxic therapy is a combination of 5 fluoro-uracil and streptozotocin, given in short courses.

In this patient, laparotomy was performed and confirmed multiple liver metastases and malignant glands at the porta hepatis. Resection was not possible. Histology and urinary indole measurements confirmed a diagnosis of carcinoid syndrome. Although still troubled by flushing and right upper quadrant pain, the patient is still alive and free of jaundice 2 years later, having had several courses of 5 FU and streptozotocin.

Case 51

Answers

1. Acute proctitis.
2. (a) Stool culture
   (b) Rectal biopsy
   (c) Barium enema.
3. (a) Sulphasalazine
   (b) Corticosteroid enemas.

Discussion

Diarrhoea and rectal bleeding accompanied by diffuse inflammation confined to the rectal mucosa indicates acute proctitis. The likeliest diagnosis in this patient is idiopathic proctitis and other causes are shown in the table. Stool cultures should always be performed in patients presenting with bloody diarrhoea. The commonest organism producing this picture in the UK is Shigella, which classically produces symptoms within 48 hours of exposure to the organism. The clinical picture is of an acute illness lasting up to 2 weeks, rather than the persistent symptoms exhibited by this

138

Table 8: Causes of an acute proctitis

Idiopathic
Infections
  Campylobacter
  Shigella
  Amoebiasis
  Gonorrhoea
  Syphilis
  Lymphogranuloma venereum
  Chlamydia
Ulcerative colitis
Crohn's disease
Drugs
  Gold
  ?Indomethacin
Chemical damage
Radiation
Trauma

patient. Another cause of infectious bloody proctitis in the UK is campylobacter infection. Recently much attention has been paid to gastrointestinal manifestations in homosexuals, where proctitis is a common problem. This has been termed the 'Gay Bowel Syndrome' and develops in promiscuous homosexuals who have a high incidence of venereal disease such as gonorrhoea, syphilis and lymphogranuloma venereum. Diagnosis depends on rectal swabs to detect Neisseria Gonorrhoea and lymphogranuloma venereum and serological tests (VDRL and fluorescent treponemal antibody test) to detect syphilis. Many are asymptomatic carriers and around 60% of patients with culture proven rectal gonorrhoea are asymptomatic and thus important reservoirs of infection, escaping recognition and treatment. Another important feature is that these patients may have more than one infection at any one time.

In idiopathic proctitis long term follow-up alone will determine whether inflammation remains confined to the rectum or will spread proximally to become ulcerative colitis. This occurs in 10% of cases and some authorities consider proctitis a localized form of ulcerative colitis. The earliest endoscopic changes in proctitis are erythema and loss of vascular pattern of the mucosa. More severe disease shows mucosal granularity and friability with contact bleeding. Advanced changes include discrete ulceration surrounded by a erythematous, friable mucosa. The microscopic appearances are similar to those of ulcerative colitis. The inflammation, unlike Crohn's disease, is confined to the mucosa (see p. 192), although in some cases clear distinction between these two conditions may not be made histologically.

The treatment of distal proctitis consists of a combination of sulphasalazine, as maintenance therapy, and topical steroids for acute exacerbations. The foam steroid enemas are easier to use and retain than liquid preparations. Some patients require high dose topical steroids or even systemic steroids to induce remission and around 10% appear resistant to all therapy. Any constipation should be treated with a high residue diet or stool bulking agents. The incidence of extra-intestinal manifestations and risk of malignancy is small compared to ulcerative colitis and thus the long term prognosis is very good.

Case 52

Answers

1. (a) Cholangiocarcinoma.
   (b) Pancreatic carcinoma.
   (c) Benign biliary stricture.
   (d) Gallstones.
2. Cholangiocarcinoma.
3. (a) Endoscopic Retrograde Cholangiopancreatography (ERCP).
   (b) Percutaneous Transhepatic Cholangiography (PTC).
   (c) Laparotomy.
4. (a) Surgical bypass, e.g. Choledochojejunostomy.
   (b) 'Stent' insertion by ERCP or PTC.

Discussion

Obstructive jaundice associated with a past history of cholecystectomy and bile duct exploration suggests a diagnosis of either recurrent biliary stones or bile duct stricture. The lack of pain during the attack of jaundice, coupled with anorexia and weight loss raise the possibility of either pancreatic carcinoma or a cholangiocarcinoma, which was the diagnosis in this case. The tumour arose in the bile ducts at the hilum of the liver and spread down the common hepatic duct but did not involve the common bile duct.

Cholangiocarcinoma is a rare tumour of unknown aetiology, but gallstones are present in about 50% of patients, and people with long-standing ulcerative colitis are 10 times more prone to develop it. The tumour often spreads sub-epithelially along the wall of the bile duct for a long distance from the obstructing mass, which makes curative resection difficult. Direct spread occurs to the hepatic artery, pancreas, duodenum and gall bladder. Over half of the patients, at the time of presentation, have direct spread or liver metastases.

The clinical features are normally not helpful in making the diagnosis since presentation is with obstructive jaundice (80%), upper abdominal pain and weight loss. It is rare though, for cholangiocarcinoma to cause clinical cholangitis and this occasionally helps differentiate it from gallstones and post-surgical biliary strictures. The abdominal ultrasound scan showing dilated intrahepatic but not extrahepatic ducts is helpful as this indicates obstruction at the liver hilum. Gallstones and carcinoma of the pancreas cause obstruction at the lower end of the common bile duct and therefore result in dilatation of both intra and extrahepatic ducts. However, cholangiocarcinoma may also arise in the distal common bile duct and in this situation ultrasound usually will not provide a definite diagnosis. At present, regardless of the site of obstruction, laparotomy plays an important role in confirming the diagnosis. The increasing availability of Percutaneous Transhepatic Cholangiography (PTC) or Endoscopic Retrograde Cholangiopancreatography (ERCP) may eventually allow pre-operative diagnosis in most cases. The latter procedure may also permit cytological and histological confirmation.

Unfortunately, curative surgical resection of cholangiocarcinoma is rarely possible. Both PTC and ERCP offer a non-surgical means of palliative treatment of jaundice and pruritus, by the insertion of a 'stent'. To insert this drainage tube a guide wire is manipulated through the tumour and then the drainage tube is passed over the guide wire. The stent should be an internal drain, that is one end above the tumour and the other end in the duodenum, which is more convenient for the patient than an external drain. In most centres surgical palliation, using one of the bypass drainage procedures discussed below still plays a major role. Regardless of the procedure performed, most patients only survive about 6 months. Other malignant lesions causing strictures of the bile ducts are carcinoma of the head of the pancreas, ampullary tumours, and rarely tumours of the duodenum. Very rarely enlarged nodes in the porta hepatis may compress the common hepatic duct. In the absence of previous biliary surgery, all biliary tract strictures should be considered malignant until proved otherwise. Ninety-seven per cent of benign biliary strictures follow surgery and other rare causes include gallstones per se. chronic pancreatitis, and sclerosing cholangitis. If there is co-existing inflammatory bowel disease, the latter is an important differential diagnosis. However, it usually results in diffuse irregularity and narrowing of the biliary tree rather than a localized stenosis.

Post-surgical biliary strictures present early if complete division of the duct has occurred, with obstructive jaundice, biliary fistula formation, or biliary peritonitis. More commonly the bile duct injury is partial and presentation is late, varying from months to years after surgery. These late strictures present with progressive but variable jaundice associated with cholangitis. If left untreated, secondary biliary cirrhosis and liver failure will develop. Although ERCP or PTC may identify the cause of biliary strictures, they are most helpful in identifying the site and extent of the obstruction so that the surgeon can plan appropriate drainage procedures.

Repair of biliary strictures must always be undertaken by a surgeon with special interest in this field, otherwise recurrence rates and mortality are high. The operation will depend on the site and length of the stricture. Where the obstruction is distal and there is adequate healthy bile duct above, a choledocho-jejunostomy is the operation of choice. With high strictures, a hepato-jejunostomy, with a Roux-en-Y limb of jejunum is created. With strictures in the hilum of the liver, even this may be difficult, necessitating dissection of a large bile duct from the left lobe of the liver and anastomosing it to the jejunum. Whatever technique is used it is important that the anastomosis is large. Prognosis of benign strictures is better if obstruction is relieved early, and if the site is distal.

Case 53

Answers

1. Caecal carcinoma.
2. Colonoscopy and biopsy.
3. (a) Adenomatous polyps.
    (b) Ulcerative colitis.

4. (a) Pulmonary disease.
   (b) Raised alkaline phosphatase (suggesting metastases).

Discussion

The most likely diagnosis is a caecal carcinoma. Carcinoma of the colon and rectum is the second most common malignancy causing death in the UK and the most common in the USA. In the UK some 17 000 people die from large bowel cancer per year (46 000 in the USA) and the majority present in the sixth and seventh decades of life. Patients may present with a variety of symptoms depending on the site of the lesion. Anaemia (75%), abdominal discomfort (55%) and weight loss (47%) are the main presenting features of caecal lesions and an abdominal mass is present in around 60%. After performing a rectal and sigmoidoscopic examination, a barium enema usually confirms the presence of a proximal carcinoma. Problems often arise however with the interpretation of equivocal filling defects in the caecum and sigmoid colon and in these instances, and in patients with diverticular disease, a colonoscopy should be performed. A number of studies have shown that colono-scopy may detect neoplastic lesions in patients with either a normal barium enema or evidence of diverticular disease. In the above patient colonoscopy confirmed the presence of a large polypoid carcinoma arising from the caecal pole.

Two pathological entities predispose to colonic cancer: adenomatous polyps and ulcerative colitis. Neoplastic polyps are the most important predisposing cause of large bowel cancer and have been found in 5–10% of asymptomatic subjects over 40 years of age. Sixty per cent of these polyps are less than 1 cm in size and around 15% greater than 2 cm. The risk of malignant change depends on: the size of the polyp, being around 40% for those over 2 cm; and its histological type, being over 40% in villous adenomas (10% of all adenomatous polyps). The evolution from a benign adenomatous polyp to cancer has been estimated to take at least 5 years and in most cases will be 10 – 15 years. Patients with familial polyposis coli or its variants, Gardner's syndrome and Turcot–Després Syndrome, often have large numbers of adenomatous polyps (average 1000) and over 80% of such patients develop colonic cancer if untreated (average age of cancer diagnosis is 40 years). Other types of polyps may also be found in the colon and rectum. The most common of these is the hyperplastic polyp which is usually located in the rectum and has no malignant potential. Hamartomatous polyps of Peutz–Jeghers Syndrome rarely involve the colon and there is no evidence that these predispose to large bowel cancer. Juvenile polyps are also hamartomata and are often encountered in young children. In juvenile polyposis large numbers of these are found in the colon and 10% of such patients may develop colorectal cancer.

It is widely accepted that patients with ulcerative colitis involving the whole colon have an increased risk of colorectal carcinoma when disease duration exceeds 10 years. Epithelial dysplasia in chronic ulcerative colitis is similar to that encountered in isolated adenomatous polyps. The main difference is that the dysplasia is more widespread and occurs in flat as well as polypoid mucosa. Unlike adenomatous polyps, pseudopolyps do not have a greater malignant potential than the surrounding flat mucosa. The precise incidence of colorectal cancer in chronic ulcerative colitis is controversial. In the UK it has been estimated that between 3 and 5% of all patients with ulcerative colitis develop large bowel cancer (5 to 10 times greater than the general population). In some American studies however, it has been reported that, after 30 years of total involvement, 50% develop malignant change.

The treatment of choice for large bowel cancer is surgical resection and some specialist units claim 90% operability with a 5 year survival of around 50%. In most regional hospitals less than 6% of colorectal cancers will be localized to the bowel wall at presentation (Duke's stage A) and two thirds will show evidence of transmural spread. Five year survival is directly related to the degree of spread and is about 90% for grade A cancer and less than 30% when regional nodes are involved. Preoperative assessment is therefore important in order to establish the presence of metastatic spread. The presence of bone pain, fractures, hepatomegaly, raised bony alkaline phosphatase and abnormal liver function tests indicate the need for further investigations such as bone scans (more sensitive than skeletal survey), ultrasound or CT liver scans and possibly tissue biopsy. In the above patient the raised alkaline phosphatase and abnormal pulmonary function tests may influence the choice of treatment. Unless associated with respiratory failure, chronic obstructive airways disease is not an absolute contraindication to surgery. After a period of intensive physiotherapy and bronchodilator therapy the majority of such patients will tolerate a general anaesthetic. The raised alkaline phosphatase may indicate bony or hepatic metastases and isoenzyme analysis is often helpful in defining its source. In the above patient the alkaline phosphatase was derived from bone and an isotope bone scan showed evidence of Paget's disease but no metastases. A right hemicolectomy was subsequently performed.

Case 54

Answers

1. Colonic obstruction due to pneumatosis coli.
2. (a) Pyloric stenosis.
   (b) Chronic obstructive airways disease.
3. (a) Broad spectrum antibiotics.
   (b) Hyperbaric oxygen.

Discussion

This patient is suffering from partial colonic obstruction as evidenced by colicky abdominal pain, gaseous distension, and fluid levels in a dilated colon on abdominal X-rays. The clinical features and investigations point to the left colon as the probable site of the obstruction. In a 60-year-old man the differential diagnosis includes a benign stricture (Diverticular disease or ischaemia) or a malignant stricture. Appendicectomy and hernia repairs rarely cause adhesions, especially after such a long interval.

The abnormal gas shadows in the left iliac fossa are suggestive of pneumatosis coli and the sigmoidoscopic appearance is typical of this condition. Pneumatosis usually occurs in patients with peptic ulcer with a degree of pyloric obstruction (60%), or chronic obstructive airways disease (30%). It may also occur in patients with scleroderma of the gastrointestinal tract, inflammatory bowel disease and ischaemic colitis. Only 2% of patients have pneumatosis without other gastrointestinal or respiratory disorders. It is thought that air enters the tissues from an ulcer crater or from a ruptured pulmonary bleb and tracks through fascial planes into the retroperitoneal space and along blood vessels into the mesentery. Recent theories implicate gas from bacterial action in the colon as the main component of the submucosal cysts. Often there are no specific symptoms but pain, partial obstruction and diarrhoea may occur. Rectal involvement produces marked tenesmus and the sigmoidoscopic appearance is typical with multiple, gas filled cysts in the submucosa appearing as bluish, sessile polyps covered by normal mucosa. Biopsy of such lesions often leads to collapse of the cyst. Small bowel involvement may produce steatorrhoea if extensive. The diagnosis is confirmed by the plain X-ray appearance of many small, discrete pockets of gas, sometimes associated with pneumoperitoneum. Barium studies show indentation of the barium column by the cysts.

Pneumatosis coli should be managed medically. The chief constituent of the gas filled cysts is nitrogen, which diffuses only slowly. Prolonged breathing of high concentrations of oxygen, producing an arterial oxygen tension of 200 – 300 mmHg, reduces the partial pressures of nitrogen and other gases in the blood and promotes diffusion of gas from the cysts (which usually disappear within a week). However, such high dose oxygen therapy must be carefully controlled in patients with chronic respiratory disease. Recently good results have been achieved using antibiotic therapy to decrease gas production by colonic micro-organisms. Surgery is indicated for frank obstruction, but pneumatosis often recurs and may become even more extensive. Our patient was treated with a broad spectrum antibiotic and his symptoms settled after 1 week.

Case 55

Answers

1. Whipple's disease.
2. (a) Barium meal and follow-through.
   (b) Jejunal biopsy.
   (c) Peripheral lymph node biopsy.
3. Prolonged, broad spectrum antibiotic therapy.

Discussion

The combination of weight loss, diarrhoea, pigmentation, pyrexia, lymphadenopathy and arthropathy are characteristic of Whipple's disease. An intestinal lymphoma with systemic spread needs to be excluded however. Jejunal biopsy will confirm Whipple's disease showing distortion of the villus pattern by a diffuse infiltration of PAS positive macrophages with a basophilic, stippled cytoplasm. In the macrophages and lamina propria, pathognomonic cytoplasmic inclusions of granules and rods may be seen. A barium follow through will delineate areas involved, usually distal duodenum and jejunum, and the lymph node biopsy may provide evidence of Whipple's as well as excluding a lymphoma.

Whipple's disease is a rare condition primarily affecting the small intestine, but systemic spread to virtually every organ in the body has been described. The bacilli and rods seen in biopsy material are thought to be involved in the pathogenesis, but a single organism has not been defined. The condition occurs sporadically and since there are no established cases of direct transmission of the illness, host susceptibility must play an important role. The foamy macrophages are specific for Whipple's disease although their role remains unclear. However, infiltration of the lamina propria with such cells hinders transport from intestinal epithelial cells to mucosal lymphatic channels. The clinical picture is of a malabsorption syndrome with fever, lymphadenopathy, pigmentation and a sero-negative arthropathy which may precede other manifestations by several years. Other organs involved include lungs, heart (many with endocarditis) and peripheral nervous system. The malabsorption produced is often severe, leading to profound abnormalities in body chemistry. A low albumin is common and a protein losing enteropathy occurs. Hepatosplenomegaly is unusual but has been described. The anaemia is usually due to iron deficiency, but a mixed type involving B_{12} or folate deficiency and a normochromic type may occur.

Treatment is with prolonged (1–2 years) broad spectrum antibiotics (usually tetracycline). The response to treatment is usually dramatic with marked resolution of symptoms within a month. Appropriate replacement therapy with iron, minerals and vitamins may be required as necessary. Prolonged antibiotic treatment is considered necessary since relapses occur after short term therapy and these can be anticipated from the reappearance of bacilli in biopsy specimens. The morphology of the intestinal mucosa can take up to 2 years to return to complete normality but the prognosis is now excellent, with 80% of patients becoming completely asymptomatic within 3 months.

Case 56

Answers

1. Acute viral hepatitis.
2. (a) Hepatitis A IgM Antibody.

(b) Hepatitis B surface antigen.
(c) Screen for other viruses (Ebstein–Barr virus/Cytomegalo-virus/Herpes simplex or varicella/Coxsackie).

Discussion

The symptoms, history of recent contact with a jaundiced girlfriend, and the ALT greater than 1000 IU/ℓ, strongly suggest acute viral hepatitis of the A, B, or non-A non-B variety. However, splenomegaly occurs in only 5–15% of such cases and the associated cervical lymphadenopathy and atypical lymphocytosis, raises the possibility of infectious mononucleosis. Chronic liver disease also causes splenomegaly and the presence of high transaminases could indicate a relapse of chronic active hepatitis. However, this is less likely because the duration of the illness is less than 6 months. The history of contact with jaundice and the ALT of over 500 IU/ℓ make alcoholic hepatitis unlikely.

The common causes of acute viral hepatitis in the UK are hepatitis A, hepatitis B, and non-A non-B hepatitis. Hepatitis A and hepatitis B are confirmed by the presence of the IgM hepatitis A antibody or hepatitis B surface antigen, respectively. The absence of these markers and negative virology for Epstein–Barr Virus (EBV), cytomegalovirus (CMV), herpes simplex and varicella viruses, and Coxsackie viruses, would support the diagnosis of non-A non-B Hepatitis. It may sometimes be difficult to differentiate between acute viral hepatitis and relapse of chronic active hepatitis. Auto-antibodies (smooth muscle and ANF may be positive in both disorders and the liver biopsy changes similar. However, in acute hepatitis the antibody titres are low, and histological changes usually resolve within 6 months.

Hepatitis A is most commonly spread by the faecal–oral route, whereas transmission of hepatitis B and non-A non-B hepatitis in the UK is usually by intravenous drug abuse or by sexual activity, especially in homosexuals. Since blood collected for transfusion is screened for hepatitis B, the commonest cause of post blood transfusion hepatitis in this country is non-A non-B Hepatitis. The clinical picture of hepatitis can vary from being asymptomatic to fulminant liver failure, but the commonest pattern is a prodromal illness with malaise, anorexia, aversion to cigarettes, nausea, and right hypochondrial discomfort. This is followed in 50% of cases by an icteric phase with jaundice, dark urine, pale stools and pruritus. The absence of rigors helps differentiate acute viral hepatitis from extrahepatic biliary obstruction. Examination often reveals tender hepatomegaly, occasionally splenomegaly and cervical lymphadenopathy. The above patient had non-A non-B hepatitis and his case illustrates one of the complications of acute viral hepatitis, namely relapse in hepatic dysfunction after apparent clinical recovery (Relapsing Hepatitis). This may be due to infection with two viruses, having different incubation periods, or excessive exercise or alcohol during the recovery period. The relapse usually resolves spontaneously. Acute Hepatitis B infection may be associated with two syndromes caused by immune complex deposition. During the prodromal phase, patients may experience polyarthritis and a maculopapular rash. During chronic hepatitis B antigenaemia a wide spread vasculitis, producing a clinical picture of Polyarteritis Nodosa, may occur. Other complications of viral hepatitis are shown in Table 9.

Table 9: Complications or sequelae of acute viral hepatitis

Relapsing hepatitis	
Fulminant hepatic failure	
Cholestatic hepatitis	
Chronic hepatitis	chronic persistent
	chronic active (not after hepatitis A)
Cirrhosis	

About 5% of patients who contract Hepatitis B become chronic carriers of the virus, but only 10% of these develop progressive liver damage. This is more likely in those patients with positive Hepatitis

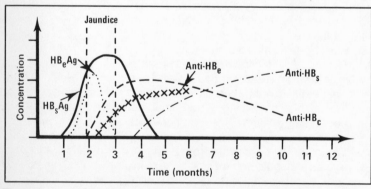

Figure 4 Serological markers of hepatitis B viral infection: appearance of antigens and antibodies to hepatitis B virus in the blood after an acute infection. (Reproduced from Sharman and Finlayson. *Diseases of the Gastrointestinal Tract and Liver*, Churchill Livingstone.)

B_e Antigen. This antigen is present when the virus is actively replicating and patients possessing it are highly infectious. The antigen and antibody responses during Hepatitis B infection are shown in Figure 4 and the clinical significance of serological findings is outlined in Table 10. (This is simply a guide and does not cover all eventualities).

Table 10: Interpretation of hepatitis B serological results

| | Highly infectious | | Low infectivity | | Resolved |
	Acute illness	Carrier	Recent acute illness	Carrier	(No risk)
HB$_s$Ag	+	+	+	+(Low Titre*)	−
HB$_e$Ag	+	+	−	−	−
Anti-HB$_c$-IgM	+/−	−	+	−	−
Anti-HB$_c$-IgG	−	+	−	+	+
Anti-HB$_s$	−	−	−	−	+
Anti-HB$_e$	−	−	+	+/−	+/−
Needle prick Transfer risk	30%		1%		0%

* i.e. the screening HEPA TEST is negative but RIA test is positive at low titre (<1:32)

Case 57

Answers

1. Sigmoid volvulus.
2. (a) Sigmoid carcinoma.
   (b) Diverticular disease.
   (c) Ischaemic colitis.
3. Barium enema.
4. (a) Decompression at sigmoidoscopy.
   (b) Surgical resection.

Discussion

The patient is suffering from a volvulus of the pelvic colon. In the UK, this condition accounts for only 9% of mechanical obstruction of the colon but it is more common in Eastern Europe, India, Scandinavia and Peru. The volvulus results from axial rotation of the pelvic colon and usually develops in patients with a redundant sigmoid loop. There is evidence that chronic ingestion of a high fibre diet may predispose to its development, males are more commonly affected than females and patients are usually middle aged or elderly. There is often a history of recurrent acute attacks of abdominal pain followed by the passage of large quantities of flatus and faeces. During these attacks the pelvic loop may rotate half to one turn with spontaneous resolution. If the loop rotates more than one to one and a half turns, venous and even arterial compression occurs producing congestion and subsequent gangrene. Abdominal distension develops very quickly due to the diffusion of CO_2 from the congested veins and after $2 - 3$ hours there is marked left sided abdominal distension. Constipation is usually absolute and if the volvulus persists generalized abdominal distension develops after 6 hours. Three other diagnoses that should be considered in this patient are an obstructing sigmoid carcinoma, complicated sigmoid diverticular disease and ischaemic colitis. However, the acute onset of pain while straining at stool and the recurrent acute attacks of pain and distension are more typical of a volvulus. In addition, patients have no weight loss, rectal bleeding or alteration in bowel habit between the attacks of volvulus.

The diagnosis is usually confirmed by the appearances of the plain abdominal X-rays. These show gross gaseous dilatation of the colon and a massively distended sigmoid, forming an inverted 'U' owing to torsion. If the plain films suggest a sigmoid colon volvulus and there is no clinical evidence of strangulation a barium enema should be performed in order to determine whether the volvulus is incomplete (180 degree turn) or complete (360+ degrees). The complete volvulus will produce a tapered narrowing of the barium column which has a 'bird's beak' appearance. Occasionally an incomplete volvulus may be reduced during the barium enema.

In patients with a sigmoid volvulus, decompression should initially be attempted using a sigmoidoscope or colonoscope. If this procedure is successful, elective surgery should be performed at a later date to prevent recurrence. If deflation does not succeed, laparotomy should be performed immediately and the sigmoid colon resected after decompression of the entire colon.

Case 58

Answers

1. Systemic sclerosis.
2. (a) Jejunal aspiration with anaerobic culture.
   (b) ^{14}C glycocholate or xylose breath test.
3. (a) Low fat diet.
   (b) Broad spectrum antibiotics.

Discussion

The combination of intestinal pseudo-obstruction, oesophageal reflux, steatorrhoea and cutaneous abnormalities strongly suggest a diagnosis of systemic sclerosis. Further questioning revealed a long history of Raynaud's phenomenon and the diagnosis was confirmed by skin biopsy.

Gastrointestinal tract abnormalities occur in 50% of patients with advanced systemic sclerosis. Of these 70% have oesophageal involvement and 40% small bowel disease. Colonic and gastric abnormalities occur much less frequently. Oesophageal involvement results in absent peristalsis of the lower two-thirds of the oesophagus and a reduced sphincter pressure. The resulting acid reflux causes oesophagitis and occasionally peptic stricture. The poor motility also predisposes to moniliasis in the oesophagus. Patients usually respond to continuous cimetidine therapy, antacids and appropriate antifungal treatment.

Small bowel involvement causes reduced motility and dilatation of the intestine (pseudo-obstruction) with associated bacterial overgrowth. In the early stages, there appears to be a defect in the cholinergic neural control of motility and at this stage, oral metoclopramide or bethanechol may stimulate contractile activity. Later on, smooth muscle atrophy occurs and these drugs are ineffective. Steatorrhoea is partly due to bacterial overgrowth and partly because of the decreased epithelial permeability produced by submucosal collagen deposition. Therefore in contrast to most cases of bacterial overgrowth serum folate may be low. The two most useful gastrointestinal investigations in this case are jejunal aspiration and ^{14}C glycocholate or xylose breath test to define the existence of bacterial overgrowth (*see* p. 113). A less specific investigation would be urinary indicans. Antibiotic therapy may partly correct malabsorption and a low fat diet, supplemented with protein and MCT oil, can help to maintain nutrition.

D-penicillamine, colchicine and corticosteroids have all been used to arrest the progress of systemic sclerosis but with disappointing results. The prognosis in those with severe gastrointestinal tract involvement is grave, as these usually have advanced disease. Our patient, although making a good initial response to parenteral nutrition, by gaining weight, feeling better and losing most of his gastrointestinal symptoms, continued to deteriorate in terms of mobility, pulmonary and renal involvement and died 2 years later.

Case 59

Answers

1. (a) Benign oesophageal stricture.
   (b) Malignant stricture.
   (c) Oesophageal motility disorder.
2. (a) Barium swallow.
   (b) Endoscopy and biopsy.
3. Endoscopic dilatation.

Discussion

The differential diagnosis in this patient is oesophageal stricture, either benign or malignant, and a motility disorder, such as achalasia or diffuse oesophageal spasm. Dysphagia, as a presenting symptom in a woman of this age, almost always has an organic basis and should be thoroughly investigated. It may be difficult to distinguish clinically between a benign and malignant stricture and distinguishing features are discussed on p. 65.

The commonest cause of a benign stricture is gastro-oesophageal reflux. Prolonged reflux oesophagitis over many years is more likely to lead to a stricture, but it has been described in patients who deny reflux symptoms or in the elderly following periods of recumbency or prolonged nasogastric intubation. Other important predisposing factors include gastrectomy, progressive systemic sclerosis and treated achalasia.

Initial investigations are designed to confirm the presence of a stricture. Barium swallow is a useful investigation and in addition to detecting a stricture will outline its size, length and possibly its nature. It is also useful in diagnosing motility disorders, which are easily missed at endoscopy. However, all patients who have strictures should have an endoscopy and biopsy to differentiate between benign and malignant lesions. A benign stricture usually looks smooth at endoscopy with evidence of oesophagitis or peptic ulceration, while a malignant stricture is irregular with polypoid projections.

Treatment of strictures depends on the cause. Strictures secondary to tablet ingestion are easily dilated by Bougienage. Strictures caused by liquid corrosives may also be dealt with in this manner but most are too long and narrow and require surgery often with replacement by colon or jejunum. Peptic strictures can be treated as for reflux oesophagitis and approximately 30% may resolve without dilatation. The remainder will require Bougienage and in many, recurrent dilatation is necessary. After the first 6 months, few patients should need more than two or three dilatations a year and it is suggested that yearly cytology and biopsy specimens should be taken because of the possibility of malignant transformation. In younger patients who may face many years of repeated Bougienage, surgery to prevent gastro-oesophageal reflux is the treatment of choice. Because of its complications, surgery is, however, not the first choice in the middle aged and elderly. Malignant strictures are difficult to treat since the carcinoma often presents at an advanced stage. Surgery is hazardous with an operative mortality of upto 20% and long term survival is only 5% at 5 years. Nevertheless, resection is the treatment of choice when tumour is localized. Palliative measures include radiotherapy and endoscopic intubation. The latter technique is rapidly gaining popularity and is now the treatment of choice for unoperable malignant strictures, giving good symptomatic improvement although not affecting the natural history of the disease.

Case 60

Answers

1. (a) Carcinoma of the pancreas.
   (b) Gallstones obstructing the common bile duct.
   (c) Tumours of biliary tract.
2. Palpable gall bladder implies gallstones are not the cause of the jaundice (Courvoisier's Law).
3. Abdominal ultrasound scan.

Discussion

The above patient had pancreatic carcinoma. The incidence of this condition is increasing and is currently around 1:10 000 of the population. Its aetiology is unknown, but cigarette smoking (twice the expected incidence) and excessive coffee intake have been implicated. Sixty to seventy per cent of tumours are located in the head of the pancreas and frequently obstruct its duct and common bile duct. The commonest presenting symptom is upper abdominal pain (63%) which may radiate into the back. Weight loss (48%) and jaundice (36%) although less frequent presenting symptoms are invariably present during the course of the disease. Occasionally patients present with diabetes mellitus or with thrombophlebitis. On examination, 40% have hepatomegaly and a similar proportion jaundice. An abdominal mass is palpable in 24% of cases and the gallbladder in 7%. The latter finding, though not frequent, is helpful in excluding gallstones (Courvoisier's Law). The exception to Courvoisier's Law is when one stone obstructs the common bile duct, and another impacts in the cystic duct (Hartmann's pouch) thereby producing a combination of jaundice and a palpable gall bladder.

The most useful diagnostic test is abdominal ultrasound or CT scanning which, in experienced hands, will detect 90% of tumours. Where this only shows dilatation of the common bile duct, the diagnosis can usually be made on PTC or ERCP. Endoscopic retrograde pancreatography may also show obstruction of the pancreatic duct and if brush cytology is performed a histological diagnosis may be made. This may also be achieved by percutaneous fine needle aspiration of the pancreatic head under ultrasonic guidance. Coeliac axis arteriography may be helpful in certain cases. Laparotomy is frequently used to confirm the diagnosis, even in specialized centres.

Unfortunately, at the time of diagnosis, most pancreatic carcinomas have spread beyond the gland and therefore palliative drainage procedures performed either at laparotomy or during ERCP or PTC are only feasible (*see* p. 140). When the tumour appears to be localized, curative resection can be attempted by performing a Whipple's operation or total pancreatectomy with splenectomy. Both operations have a mortality of up to 20% and 5 year survival is only 5 – 10%. The overall survival for carcinoma of the pancreas is less than 1% at 5 years.

3 Normal Laboratory Values

Haematology

Haemoglobin	♂	13.5–18.0 g/dl
	♀	11.5–16.5 g/dl
ESR	♂	1–10 mm/hour
	♀	1–15 mm/hour
MCH		27–32 pg
MCHC		32–36 g/dl
MCV		76–96 fl
Platelets		$150–400 \times 10^9/\ell$
WBC	Total	$4.0–11.0 \times 10^9/\ell$
	Neutrophils	$2.7–7.5 \times 10^9/\ell$ (40–75%)
	Lymphocytes	$1.5–3.5 \times 10^9/\ell$ (20–45%)
	Monocytes	$0.2–0.8 \times 10^9/\ell$ (2–10%)
	Eosinophils	$0.04–0.44 \times 10^9/\ell$ (1–6%)
Prothrombin Time		10–14 seconds
Folate	Serum	4.0–18.0 μg/ℓ
	RBC	87–337 μg/ℓ
Vitamin B_{12}		170–1000 ng/ℓ

Biochemistry

Blood

Sodium		135–145 mmol/ℓ
Potassium		3.3–5.3 mmol/ℓ
Bicarbonate		24–34 mmol/ℓ
Creatinine		60–120 μmol/ℓ
Urea		2.5–7.5 mmol/ℓ
Glucose	Fasting	3.0–6.4 mmol/ℓ
	Non-fasting	3.5–10.3 mmol/ℓ
Total Protein		62–82 g/ℓ
Albumin		35–50 g/ℓ
ALT		5–30 IU/ℓ
AST		5–45 IU/ℓ
Gamma GT	♂	10–43 IU/ℓ
	♀	7–31 IU/ℓ
Alkaline Phosphatase		30–130 IU/ℓ
Bilirubin	Total	1—20 μmol/ℓ
	Conjugated	0–5 μmol/ℓ
Corrected Calcium		2.1–2.6 mmol/ℓ
Amylase		< 300 IU/ℓ
Iron		11–32 μmol/ℓ
TIBC		45–70 μmol/ℓ
Immunoglobulins	IgA	0.9–4.5 g/ℓ
	IgG	6.0–18.0 g/ℓ
	IgM	0.5–2.2 g/ℓ

Faecal

Weight	< 200 g/day
Osmolality	<350 m. osm/kg
pH	5.85–8.45
Fat	< 18 mmol/day

Urine

Xylose	>23% of a 5g dose in 5 hours

Miscellaneous

Wedged hepatic venous pressure   up to 5 mmHg

Schirmer's Test: Normal   > 10 mm
                    Borderline   5–10 mm } over 5 minutes
                    Abnormal   < 5 mm

Part 2

Reviews

Management of Peptic Ulcer Disease

Peptic ulcer disease is a common condition affecting about 1 in every 5 men and 1 in 10 women in the UK, at some time in their lives. Duodenal ulcer occurs 2–3 times more frequently than gastric ulcer.

Diagnosis of Peptic Ulcer

The history and physical examination are unreliable indicators of peptic ulcer disease and have little value in predicting whether an ulcer is gastric or duodenal. Thus accurate diagnosis relies on radiological or endoscopic visualization of the upper gastrointestinal tract. Endoscopy is far more accurate than barium meal (single and double contrast) and detects over 95% of peptic ulcers. The existence of a scarred duodenum on the barium meal does not indicate active ulceration and superficial ulcers may be missed in around 20% of cases. Although a barium meal may show the presence of a gastric ulcer, it is often difficult to distinguish between benign and malignant ulceration. Gastroscopy with 4 – 6 biopsies from the gastric ulcer margin may distinguish benign and malignant disease in over 90% of cases and the addition of cytology may increase the yield to around 95%. Thus gastroscopy is the procedure of choice in investigating patients presenting with dyspepsia.

Initial Treatment of Benign Ulcers

The initial management of benign gastric ulcer and duodenal ulcer is similar and based on the concept that ulceration develops from an imbalance between damaging intraluminal factors, such as acid, and the protective properties of surface epithelium. Thus most of the available drugs either reduce acid secretion or enhance mucosal defence mechanisms. Despite these different modes of action most drugs heal about 80% of acute peptic ulcers.

1. Drugs which reduce gastric acidity

Various antacids have been used for decades to relieve peptic ulcer symptoms. In conventional doses relatively little acid is neutralized and the antacid is quickly emptied from the stomach. Such regimens do not heal peptic ulcers. In large doses (around 500 ml/day) antacids may heal ulcers but in the UK such treatment is unpopular with patients. Acid secretion may be inhibited by a variety of drugs. Anticholinergics were initially used but found to have unacceptable side effects. Newer anticholinergic drugs, such as pirenzepine, are more effective in healing ulcers and appear to have slightly less side-effects than the first generation drugs. The discovery of histamine H_2 receptor antagonists has revolutionized ulcer healing and the two most popular drugs, cimetidine and ranitidine, heal over 80% of peptic ulcers over a 6 – 8 week period, with minimal side effects. Such drugs may also cause temporary healing of malignant ulceration and therefore symptomatic response to such drugs should not be used as a criterion for distinguishing benign from malignant ulcers.

2. Drugs which enhance mucosal defence mechanisms

A number of drugs have been shown to heal peptic ulcers by mechanisms which are independent of acid secretion. The first of these was carbenoxolone and although this heals around 80% of gastric and duodenal ulcers, it has serious aldosterone-like side-effects such as hypertension, oedema and hypokalaemia. Another extract from liquorice, 'Caved S', has very little aldosterone activity and has recently been shown to heal a similar proportion of peptic ulcers. The precise mechanism of action of these drugs remains unknown but effects on mucus production, cell exfoliation and non-parietal alkaline secretion may be of importance. A number of other drugs also heal ulcers by effects on mucosal defence, including colloidal bismuth, 'sucralfate', and prostaglandins. In various clinical trials all these agents appear to heal about 80–90% of peptic ulcers over a 4–8 week period and are remarkably free of side-effects. In the UK, prostaglandin E_2 analogues are not yet available for routine clinical use.

Follow-up and Ulcer Relapse

Patients with gastric ulcer require endoscopy at 6 – 8 weeks to confirm ulcer healing and exclude gastric malignancy. If the ulcer has not healed, treatment may be continued for a further 4 – 6 weeks, provided biopsies (and cytology) reveal no malignancy. Failure of ulcer healing at this time may necessitate either surgery or trial of a different drug, depending largely on the age and general health of the patient. Duodenal ulcers are invariably benign and healing at the end of 6 – 8 weeks treatment, can usually be inferred from the symptomatic response. If symptoms persist endoscopy is indicated to determine whether they are due to an active ulcer. Failure of ulcer healing may be managed by continued treatment for another 6 weeks or changing to another drug. In some patients cigarette smoking may be responsible for the poor response; ulcer healing in smokers being significantly less than in matched non-smokers. Other factors such as alcohol and analgesic intake (e.g. aspirin) do not appear to modify ulcer healing. If duodenal ulcers persist despite an adequate 3 month treatment period, serum gastrin should be measured to exclude the Zollinger–Ellison Syndrome and if normal, patients referred for surgical therapy.

Following initial ulcer healing, approximately 60 – 80% of patients will experience a relapse within 12 – 18 months and patients with duodenal ulcer may, on average, expect 1 or 2 relapses per year. If patients are placed on 'maintenance' therapy with low doses of cimetidine (400 mg nocte) or ranitidine (150 mg nocte) this relapse rate may be significantly reduced to approximately 20%. Unfortunately, when such maintenance therapy is discontinued, relapses occur and the natural history of the disease is unaltered. Thus for duodenal ulcers that relapse once or twice per year, 4 – 6 week treatment courses are recommended for each symptomatic relapse or surgery considered. A similar regimen applies to relapsing gastric ulcers, although endoscopic confirmation (plus biopsy) of relapse should be obtained. Long term maintenance therapy for gastric or duodenal ulcer should be restricted to those in whom ulcer relapse has resulted in gastrointestinal bleeding or perforation and who are unsuitable or unwilling to have surgical therapy, and those with frequent relapses (more than 4 per year), who do not wish surgery. Until the safety of long term treatment with H_2 receptor antagonists has been established, other patients should be treated with intermittent 4 – 6 week courses.

Medical versus Surgical Therapy

In contrast to medical therapy, surgery offers a patient the prospect of 'cure' rather than suppression of ulcer activity. Unfortunately, this is at the expense of permanent alteration to gastroduodenal anatomy and can give rise to abdominal symptoms which may be as disabling as ulcer manifestations. In an uncomplicated ulcer, the response to medical therapy and need for surgery is impossible to predict at initial presentation. The majority of patients with benign peptic ulcers are quite happy to receive medical treatment when ulcer relapse occurs. If, however, for socio-economic reasons the patient wishes a more permanent solution, surgery should be advocated when relapse occurs. The development of perforation or recurrent gastrointestinal bleeding are clear indications for surgery. In patients with haemorrhage, a trial of 12 months maintenance therapy may be worth considering, with referral for surgery if bleeding subsequently returns during ulcer relapse. Patients with recurrent gastric ulcer should be offered surgery earlier than those with duodenal ulcer because they are on average 10–15 years older and tend to tolerate complications, such as haemorrhage, less well. The proportion of duodenal ulcer patients requiring surgery is less than 1 in 10 and the majority are a result of 'failed medical therapy'. Of all patients referred for peptic ulcer surgery, 80% have a satisfactory result. The remainder continue to suffer from abdominal symptoms related to postgastric surgery syndromes (*see* p. 163) or to recurrent or unhealed ulcer.

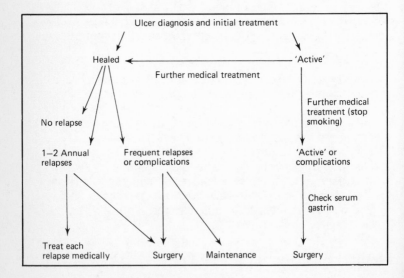

Figure 5 Medical management of peptic ulcers

Post-Surgical Syndromes

Oesophagus

Anti-Reflux Surgery

A variety of surgical procedures have been used to prevent acid reflux and several post-operative syndromes are recognized. Gas-bloat or 'the post-fundoplication syndrome', due to 'supercontinence' of the lower oesophageal sphincter, results in post-prandial fullness, abdominal bloating and inability to belch or vomit. It occurs in approximately 10% of patients but is distressing in less than 5%. Damage to vagal fibres at operation may cause dilatation of the oesophagus, diarrhoea and gas-bloat symptoms in 3% of patients – the so-called 'denervation syndrome'. Symptoms may be alleviated by pyloroplasty. Dysphagia may occur in 10 – 15% of patients but usually resolves within 4 months. Recurrence of reflux may occur if sutures tear through the cuff of stomach used to secure the fundus below the diaphragm, or when the cuff slips allowing the oesophagus to 'telescope'.

Myotomy

Myotomy of the lower oesophageal sphincter almost always abolishes dysphagia when performed for achalasia, but produces distressing oesophageal reflux in 20–40% of patients. Recurrent dysphagia may be due to incomplete myotomy or peptic stricture formation.

Stomach

Many of the sequelae of vagotomy and drainage also occur after partial gastrectomy and for convenience both types of surgery will be discussed together.

Delayed gastric emptying and reflux

Dysphagia and gastro-oesophageal reflux occur after vagotomy or partial gastrectomy and usually improve rapidly with time. Delayed gastric emptying is unusual after gastric surgery but may occur early due to oedema of the anastomosis, or late as a result of recurrent ulcer, fibrotic scarring of the anastomosis or gastroparesis.

In the absence of any demonstrable mechanical obstruction ('Post-vagotomy gastroparesis'), metoclopramide or a cholinergic agent may be helpful.

Increased duodeno-gastric reflux of bile occurs after all operations for peptic ulcer and may result in bile vomiting and epigastric discomfort. Symptoms occur in up to 15% of patients soon after operation, but improve with the passage of time. Cholestyramine, hydrotalcite and aludrox all bind bile salts but are disappointing in clinical practice. Metoclopramide, by speeding gastric emptying, may be helpful. In severe cases the construction of a Roux-en-Y loop may be necessary to prevent bile reflux. Gastritis possibly secondary to bile reflux occurs in 60–100% of patients after partial gastrectomy, especially around the anastomosis, but in most patients is asymptomatic.

Gastric Incontinence (dumping)

Symptoms due to gastric incontinence occur in 10–30% of patients after vagotomy and drainage, and are severe in 5% but incapacitating in <1%. Lower incidences occur after proximal gastric vagotomy (PGV) (1–6%) and symptoms are rarely severe. Incidence after partial gastrectomy varies between 15–40%. Symptoms occur 10–20 minutes after a meal (early dumping) due to rapid emptying of osmotically active sugars and polysaccharides into the small bowel. These attract large volumes of fluid into the gut lumen resulting in distension with consequent abdominal fullness, nausea and colic. The large bolus of fluid also precipitates diarrhoea, and a variety of other systemic symptoms occur such as weakness, faintness, drowsiness, palpitations and sweating. Tachycardia, hypotension and ECG changes may also occur. The exact cause of these symptoms is unknown but neural and hormonal factors (e.g. 5HT release) have been suggested as well as hypovolaemia. 'Late' dumping occurs 90–120 minutes after a meal and is due to excess output of insulin in response to a rapid peak in blood glucose.

As symptoms improve with time, many patients require no specific treatment. Avoidance of refined carbohydrate or starchy foods and frequent small, dry meals are advocated. Insulin or tolbutamide before meals are of limited value and serotonin antagonists have not been properly evaluated. Ingestion of Guar gum to delay absorption, and dissaccharidase inhibitors to delay digestion have also been used but further studies are required to confirm their value. Conversion of a Billroth II gastrectomy to a Billroth I may help in severe cases and antiperistaltic loops of small bowel have been tried with variable results.

Post-vagotomy Diarrhoea

This problem rarely occurs after PGV (1–8%) but affects 20–30% of patients undergoing vagotomy and drainage procedures. It is severe in 10% and intractable in 1%. Diarrhoea may be continuous or intermittent, occurring in explosive attacks, and both patterns improve during the first few months after operation. Many factors may contribute to the diarrhoea such as gastric incontinence, motility disturbances, altered gut flora and alterations in bile salt absorption and secretion. Vagotomy or partial gastrectomy may also reveal previously latent conditions such as coeliac disease, lactose intolerance or IgA deficiency. Medical treatments include antidiarrhoeal drugs and cholestyramine, and in severe cases reconstructive surgery or a reversed peristaltic loop may be attempted. Cholecystectomy usually aggravates post-vagotomy diarrhoea and this combination of operations should be avoided if possible.

Metabolic Sequelae

Mild malabsorption may occur after gastric surgery (faecal fat <35 mmol) but this is usually of little clinical significance. Anaemia occurs in about 40% of patients, 15 years after operation, and iron deficiency is the commonest cause (decreased intake, reduced absorption and occult bleeding). Low Vitamin B_{12} levels occur in 14% of post-gastrectomy patients, secondary to intrinsic factor deficiency, but megaloblastic anaemia is uncommon. Weight loss is common after gastric surgery due mainly to reduced calorie intake, but occasionally aggravated by slight malabsorption.

Miscellaneous

Recurrent ulcers occur in 5–10% of patients after vagotomy or Billroth I gastrectomy but in only 1% after Billroth II gastrectomy. Hypergastrinaemia should be excluded and medical treatment tried before considering re-operation.

Carcinoma of the stomach occurs in 1–3% of partial gastrectomy patients after 15 years, mainly at the anastomotic site. Although evidence is conflicting, gastric surgery probably increases the risk of developing gastric carcinoma in the stomach remnant.

The afferent loop syndrome was thought to be due to the accumulated bile in the afferent loop being suddenly emptied into the stomach through the stoma resulting in bilious vomiting. Most of these patients were however misdiagnosed and were suffering from duodenogastric reflux. Rarely, acute afferent loop obstruction occurs and requires urgent surgical correction.

Small Intestine

Small Bowel Resection

Short segments of small intestine can be resected without causing disability because of the large functional reserve in absorptive capacity. Problems may however occur after large resections, after removal of the terminal ileum which has specific absorptive functions, or when the remaining small intestine or colon is abnormal. The normal length of small bowel is variable and, therefore, the percentage of bowel resected is more relevant than the actual length removed. In general, if the remaining bowel is normal, resection of more than 50% will cause a degree of malabsorption, and if this exceeds 75%, special management will be required. The state of the bowel remaining after resection is important, since extensive Crohn's disease or systemic sclerosis will further reduce absorptive capacity. The presence of an intact and normal colon is also important as it may absorb up to 6 ℓ of fluid a day. Resections or disease involving the colon (especially the right side where most fluid absorption occurs) as well as the small bowel, cause greater functional loss. Resection of the ileo-caecal valve may predispose to bacterial overgrowth in the distal small bowel or result in shorter transit time, thereby reducing absorption. Concomitant heart or liver disease, or undiagnosed lactose intolerance may further aggravate the situation.

Over a period of months or years the remaining small bowel may 'adapt' leading to increased calibre, length and villous size. The stimulus to 'adaptation' is not known but luminal nutrients appear to be important as bypassed small intestine tends to undergo villous atrophy, even when associated with massive resection.

Gastric hypersecretion occurs in 50% of patients after extensive small bowel resection. The mechanism is uncertain but both fasting and meal stimulated serum gastrin levels may be elevated. A gastrin inhibitor may be removed by the resection or alternatively clearance of gastrin by the small bowel may be reduced. The large volumes of gastric juice produced increase the fluid load entering the small bowel and hyperacidity in the gut lumen contributes to malabsorption (cf Zollinger–Ellison Syndrome).

Terminal Ileal Resection

Although the major absorptive area of the intestine is situated in the proximal one quarter of the small bowel, resection of jejunum can be partially compensated for by increased ileal absorption. The terminal ileum, however, has specific absorptive functions which cannot be achieved by other parts of the small bowel. Vitamin B_{12} and bile salts are mainly absorbed in the terminal ileum. Bile salt malabsorption, due to ileal resection or dysfunction, allows bile acids to enter the colon and inhibit colonic absorption, while enhancing secretion of water and electrolytes. Bile salts also increase colonic motility and the combined effect results in a secretory diarrhoea (see p. 189). Increased hepatic synthesis may initially compensate for the loss of bile salts. However ileal resections in excess of 100 cm lead to a reduction in the circulating bile salt pool and decreased concentrations in the duodenal lumen after eating. When this concentration is less than the critical micellar concentration, malabsorption of fat occurs with steatorrhoea. In addition, reduction of the bile acid pool leads to lithogenic bile and this explains the increased incidence of gallstones in patients who have had terminal ileal resection or disease.

Short Bowel Syndrome

A combination of any or all of the above mechanisms may be responsible for the manifestations of the short bowel syndrome. During the first few days and weeks following massive small bowel resection, severe watery diarrhoea may occur resulting in dehydration, electrolyte imbalance and acid-base disturbances. Multiple vitamin and mineral deficiencies may also develop leading to anaemia, tetany, osteomalacia and neuropathy.

Patients often require prolonged total parenteral nutrition with gradual introduction of oral feeding using small frequent meals and appropriate mineral and vitamin supplementation. A low fat diet with MCT oil and carbohydrate restriction may be useful. H_2 receptor antagonists reduce gastric hypersection though they are rarely needed in the long term, and antidiarrhoeal agents like loperamide may reduce stool frequency. Oxalate from dietary sources is absorbed from the colon and this is increased in the presence of steatorrhoea, producing hyperoxaluria and increased incidence of renal stones. Several possible mechanisms exist; fatty acids in the gut lumen may combine with calcium to form calcium soaps leaving less calcium to combine with oxalate. The resulting oxalates are more soluble and thus easily absorbed. In addition bile salts and long chain fatty acids may increase colonic mucosal permeability to oxalate. A low oxalate diet and calcium supplements are useful therapeutic measures in these patients. Further surgery should be avoided if at all possible as vagotomy, gastrectomy or further resections of small bowel, will all aggravate the above problems. The

168

construction of antiperistaltic loops of small bowel to slow transit rarely prove useful.

Jejuno-Ileal Bypass

This operation has a mortality of 5% and many severe side effects. By its very nature severe malabsorption, weight loss, and a large blind loop is produced.

Early Complications (0–2 months post-operatively)

Frequent bowel actions with loose stools occur in all patients but may settle to 3 or 4 loose stools a day within a few months. Patients with persistent troublesome diarrhoea may be helped by a low fat diet. Occasionally such symptoms are so severe as to require restoration of normal bowel continuity. Electrolyte, mineral and vitamin derangements may be corrected by appropriate replacement therapy.

Intermediate Complications (3 months – 2 years (post-operatively)

Increased incidences of oxalate renal stones and gallstones occur as in patients with ileal resection and are managed in the same way. Colonic pseudo-obstruction occurs in 5% of patients and pneumatosis intestinalis in 10%.

Most obese patients have fatty infiltration of the liver and this increases during the first 3 months post-operatively, as triglycerides, mobilized during the rapid weight loss phase, are stored in the liver. The infiltration gradually resolves and in most patients is not associated with symptoms or hepatic dysfunction (apart from raised transaminases). In 5% of patients, however, progressive liver disease associated with vomiting, persistent diarrhoea, jaundice and liver failure develops. Liver biopsy shows changes indistinguishable from acute alcoholic hepatitis and if patients survive long enough, cirrhosis develops. The cause of this deterioration may be protein calorie malnutrition and if oral or IV nutrition does not correct the abnormalities, urgent restoration of intestinal anatomy should be performed.

Late Complications (more than 2 years post-operatively)

Excessive weight loss is rare (0.5%) but may require re-operation to shorten the bypassed loop. More commonly (10%) patients have insufficient weight loss as the functioning bowel hypertrophies. Late deficiencies in vitamin B_{12}, Ca^{2+} and Vitamin D etc should be avoided by appropriate monitoring. Psychiatric problems are not uncommon but may stem from pre-existing psychiatric disorders.

Blind Loop Syndrome

This has been discussed in detail elsewhere (*see* p. 112).

Colon

Partial Colectomy

Under normal circumstances the colon actively absorbs sodium and water and has a large functional reserve. When fluid entering the colon is increased (as in small bowel disease) the absorbing capacity of the colon may be exceeded. Right-sided colonic resection when combined with terminal ileal resection may cause diarrhoea. Patients are more vulnerable to the effects of various diarrhoeal diseases after colonic resection, because of the smaller functional reserve of the remaining colon. Left sided resection rarely causes problems.

Anorectal Surgery

The main problems following anorectal surgery are incontinence and sexual dysfunction. Sexual dysfunction occurs in up to two-thirds of patients undergoing wide excision of the rectum and this is permanent in one-third. In non-malignant conditions strenuous efforts to avoid damage to the pelvic nerves at operation will minimize this problem. Anorectal procedures, such as anal dilatation and haemorrhoidectomy, cause minor defects of continence but unless there is major damage to the anal sphincters this is not clinically significant. Patients with minor defects of continence are, however, more prone to episodes of incontinence when afflicted by diarrhoeal illnesses.

Biliary Tract

Post-cholecystectomy Syndrome

This vague term is used to describe a variety of symptoms after cholecystectomy. Mild symptoms such as dyspepsia, diarrhoea and upper abdominal discomfort occur in about 30%. Severe symptoms of colic, cholangitis and biliary leakage occur less frequently. Half of all patients with post-cholecystectomy symptoms have demonstrable organic disease either related to the biliary tract (e.g. retained CBD stones or papillary stenosis) or pre-existing conditions mistakenly attributed to biliary tract disease (e.g. oesophagitis peptic ulcer, pancreatic disease). Motility disorders of the biliary tree after cholecystectomy rarely explain post-cholecystectomy symptoms but functional disorders like irritable bowel syndrome should be considered. Cystic duct remnants are unlikely to be symptomatic unless stones are present.

Post-operative Jaundice

There are many causes of post-operative hyperbilirubinaemia as illustrated in Table 11.

Table 11: Causes of post-operative jaundice

Early
Surgical handling of liver
Benign post-operative jaundice
Halothane hepatitis or other drug-induced
Post-operative pancreatitis
Haemolysis
Sepsis
Decompensation of pre-existing liver disease
Portal vein thrombosis
Resolving haematoma
Gilbert's Syndrome

Late
Scarring of bile ducts
Cholangitis
Biliary fistula
Viral hepatitis

Investigation of Jaundice

A number of disorders may result in jaundice and the most common are summarized in Table 12.

While most cases of post-hepatic jaundice need prompt surgical relief, patients with prehepatic and hepatic jaundice may be harmed by inappropriate surgery. It is therefore vital that this distinction is made at an early stage.

A careful history and physical examination will differentiate 'surgical' from 'medical' jaundice in around 80% of cases. The patient's age is an important factor, with viral hepatitis being the commonest cause of the jaundice in the second and third decades of life and gallstones and neoplasia become progressively more common over the age of 40 years. A positive family history suggests an inherited defect in bilirubin transport or a haemoglobinopathy. Contact with jaundice or blood transfusion within the last 6 months, recent injections and drug abuse, or homosexual activities suggest viral hepatitis. Recent travel abroad may indicate an infective aetiology. An accurate drug and alcohol history is also essential. Weight loss, especially with progressive jaundice, favours malignancy. Jaundice with pale stools, dark urine, and pruritus implies cholestasis and if such symptoms are associated with abdominal pain, fever, and rigors then extrahepatic obstruction is likely. A history of previous operations on the biliary tree or pancreas, raises the possibility of a biliary stricture.

On examination, the degree of jaundice can be helpful. Mild jaundice, in conjunction with splenomegaly, suggests haemolysis

Table 12: Disorders which may result in jaundice

Pre-Hepatic	
Increased bilirubin production	Haemolysis
Hepatic	
Inherited defects in bilirubin transport	Gilbert's Syndrome
	Crigler–Najjar Syndrome
	Dubin–Johnson Syndrome
	Viral hepatitis
	Alcoholic hepatitis
Hepatocellular damage	Drug-induced hepatitis
	Cirrhosis
	Chronic active hepatitis
	Drug-induced
Intrahepatic biliary cholestasis	Cholestasis of pregnancy
	Primary biliary cirrhosis
Post-Hepatic	
	Gallstones
	Pancreatitis
Obstruction to	Neoplasia
biliary tree	Benign biliary strictures
	Sclerosing cholangitis

while marked and progressive jaundice favours obstruction of a large bile duct. Stigmata of chronic liver disease, particularly spider naevi, usually indicate a form of cirrhosis. A palpable gall bladder suggests common bile duct obstruction, usually from pancreatic carcinoma (Courvoisier's Law). The presence of ascites is indicative of either malignant disease or cirrhosis. A large irregular liver may result from either of these conditions but if splenomegaly is present, cirrhosis is more likely.

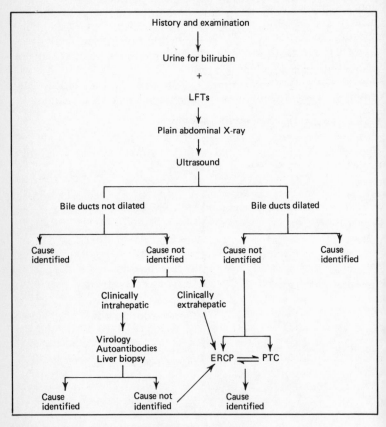

Figure 6 Clinical assessment of a jaundiced patient

Liver function tests per se are not reliable in differentiating between extrahepatic and hepatic causes of jaundice. However, cholestatic liver function tests with bilirubinuria exclude Gilbert's Syndrome and haemolysis. Once a prehepatic cause is excluded, a plain abdominal X-ray may identify calcified gall stones or calcific pancreatitis. If negative, an abdominal ultrasound scan is the next investigation of choice as it is non-invasive, comparatively cheap, available in most hospitals, and will differentiate accurately between 'surgical' and 'medical' jaundice in over 90% of cases ('surgical' cases being identified by dilatation of the bile ducts). However it is dependent on operator skill and is less reliable when there is mild jaundice (48% success if bilirubin is < 200 μmol/ℓ). Ascites, excess fat or intestinal gas also reduce accuracy. Computerized tomography (CT Body Scan) is at least as accurate as ultrasound scanning, but is more costly and less available. If bile ducts are dilated but the scan has not defined the cause, a Percutaneous Transhepatic Cholangiogram (PTC) or Endoscopic Retrograde Cholangiopancreatography (ERCP) should be performed. Theoretically, in the presence of dilated bile ducts, PTC is preferred as the ducts should be easily entered. However, the procedure used will largely depend upon local resources and expertise, whether coagulation is normal and whether ascites is present (the latter two conditions being a relative contraindication to PTC). The therapeutic potential of ERCP should also be considered since gallstones may be removed during this procedure. Endoscopic retrograde cholangiography with stone extraction is the treatment of choice in elderly patients (more than 70 years old) who have undergone previous cholecystectomy or in patients with co-existing cardiorespiratory disease, since mortality is lower for endoscopic sphincterotomy than for surgery. Malignant strictures of the biliary system can be palliatively drained by inserting a stent (cannula) through the tumour to allow free bile drainage. This can be carried out by PTC or ERCP, but a blocked stent can only be removed and replaced by ERCP. If one procedure does not successfully outline the biliary tree and provide diagnosis the other procedure should be tried. Laparoscopy is of limited value in the investigation of obstructive jaundice.

If an ultrasound scan does not show dilated bile ducts, bile duct obstruction is not necessarily excluded. In this case it should be decided on clinical grounds whether a hepatic or extrahepatic cause is most likely. If a hepatic lesion is favoured and no hepatic abnormality has been identified on the scan, virology, autoantibodies, and liver biopsy should be performed. When extrahepatic obstruction is thought likely, an ERCP is the investigation of choice.

Liver Failure

Liver failure reflects functional abnormality of the liver rather than any specific pathological entity. It can complicate almost any form of liver disease, both acute and chronic, and in the UK, the common causes are cirrhosis, drug-induced liver damage and viral hepatitis. The clinical picture of liver failure develops when hepatic function is so impaired as to produce encephalopathy, ascites and peripheral oedema, coagulation defect or impaired immune response to infection (*see Table 13*).

Table 13: Liver functions and resultant defects in liver failure

Function	Outcome in liver failure
Protein metabolism	
Production of albumin	Ascites and peripheral oedema
Deamination of amino acids and	Hepatic encephalopathy
nitrogenous compounds	Low urea
Production of clotting factors	Coagulation defects*
Production of α and β globulins	Impaired response to infection
Vitamin K	
Stored in and used by liver	Coagulation defects*
to make clotting factors V, VII, IX, X	
Carbohydrate metabolism	
Glycogenesis	Hyperglycaemia
Gluconeogenesis	Hypoglycaemia*
Hormone metabolism	
Insulin	Hypoglycaemia*
Oestrogen/testosterone	Hypogonadism and gynaecomastia
Corticosteroids	Atrophic skin

* associated with acute hepatocellular necrosis

Hepatic Encephalopathy

Toxins derived from bacterial action on urea (80%) and non-urea protein (20%) seem to be particularly important in altering cerebral function, and reducing the intestinal protein content reverses the encephalopathy. Under normal conditions toxins absorbed from the intestine are removed by the liver before they enter the general circulation. In cirrhosis, toxins bypass the liver via porta-systemic communications while in acute, fulminant liver failure toxins are not extracted by damaged hepatocytes. Various agents have been incriminated including ammonia and derivatives of aromatic amino acids; all of which are usually elevated in blood and CSF of patients with hepatic encephalopathy. In the CNS these substances are metabolized either to normal neurotransmitters or to compounds which act as false neurotransmitters. For instance, the neurotransmitter serotonin, which is derived from the amino acid tryptophan, has been reported to be elevated. Possible false neurotransmitters are glutamine derived from ammonia and octopamine derived from amino acids. Most cases of hepatic encephalopathy result from an increased protein load, the commonest cause (29%) being uraemia (50% of these being diuretic induced). Gastrointestinal bleeding accounts for 18% of cases, 10% are related to excess oral nitrogen intake, 3% to constipation and 3% to infection, increasing amino acid catabolism. Causes unrelated to an increased protein load include: drugs (24%), particularly sedatives, tranquilizers, anaesthetics and opiate analgesics; hypokalaemic alkalosis (10%), and alcohol.

The manifestations of hepatic encephalopathy are numerous with reduced conscious level, impaired cerebration, flapping tremor (asterixis), foetor hepaticus, and constructional dyspraxia (slow and inaccurate copying of diagrams of clocks or five pointed stars) being the most common. The degree of encephalopathy can be graded as follows:

Grade I	Altered Mood – euphoria/depression – slow cerebration
Grade II	Inappropriate Behaviour Drowsiness and slurred speech
Grade III	Asleep but rouseable
Grade IV	Unresponsive except to pain
Grade V	Completely unresponsive

The management of hepatic encephalopathy begins with identification and correction of the precipitating cause. Rectal examination for melaena or constipation, clinical assessment and laboratory screen for infection, urea and electrolytes and a review of drug therapy should be performed. A low protein (20 g), high carbohydrate diet is given. Intestinal protein metabolism is reduced by giving oral Neomycin (1 g t.d.s.) to inhibit ammonia forming bacteria. Lactulose is often given in addition to neomycin although there is no clear evidence that the combination is better than either agent alone. Lactulose causes an osmotic purge, suppresses ammonia forming bacteria and prevents the ionization of non-absorbable ammonium to absorbable ammonia. The dose of lactulose required varies between 10–30 mls t.d.s.; the ideal dose being that which produces two semi-solid stools per day. If the patient is too drowsy to take oral drugs, magnesium sulphate or lactulose enemas can be given.

Ascites

The commonest cause of non-malignant ascites is cirrhosis. Impaired liver function results in hypoalbuminaemia and reduced plasma oncotic pressure, while portal hypertension increases the hydrostatic pressure. Consequently fluid enters the peritoneal cavity from splanchnic capillaries resulting in hypovolaemia and secondary hyperaldosteronism. There is usually no precipitating factor other than deteriorating liver function. Acute intestinal bleeding resulting in hypoperfusion of the liver may produce temporary impairment of liver function and subsequent ascites. In the absence of gastrointestinal bleeding, rapidly developing ascites may be due to infection, portal vein thrombosis or tumour invasion of the portal vein.

The initial investigation of ascites is a diagnostic tap (20–40 ml). The ascites is inspected for blood staining (tuberculosis or hepatocellular carcinoma) and cloudiness (Chylous or bacterial infection). Fluid is sent for cytology, culture and protein concentration. Protein levels above 30 g/ℓ (exudate) favour a malignant or inflammatory cause for the ascites.

A low sodium diet (20 mmol/day) alone is effective in reducing ascites in 20% of cases. In the absence of hepatic encephalopathy, a high protein intake is given to improve albumin synthesis. Most cases will also need diuretics and, as secondary hyperaldosteronism is usually present, spironolactone is the initial drug of choice. The initial dose is 100–200 mg/day and this may need to be increased to 400 mg daily. However, as spironolactone is not fully active until 48–72 hours after intake, the dose should not be increased too rapidly. Because the maximum volume of ascites that can be transferred from the peritoneal cavity back into the circulation is approximately 900 ml/day it is important not to produce too large a diuresis as this will merely induce pre-renal failure. The patient should be weighed daily and loss should be around 0.5 kg/day. If daily weight loss is more than 1 kg, the diuretic dose should be reduced or the drug stopped. If the weight loss is under 0.5 kg/day on a dose of 400 mg of spironolactone, frusemide (40 mg/day) may be added. Loop and thiazide diuretics are more likely to precipitate renal failure and electrolyte imbalance, and special care should be taken to monitor the clinical and electrolyte response to these agents. Paracentesis should only be performed to relieve cardio-respiratory embarrassment, since it may cause hypovolaemia with subsequent renal failure and further impairment of liver function. If ascites appears to be resistant to this regime, sodium intake and drug compliance should be checked. Sodium may inadvertently be taken in the form of drugs (e.g. parenteral penicillin and antacids), biscuits, sauces, or preservatives. If ascites is genuinely resistant, then ascitic drainage and re-infusion using a Rhodiascit filter may be performed. In patients who reaccumulate ascites or who are non-compliant with their therapy, a Le Veen shunt may be inserted. Both Rhodiascit and Le Veen shunts should not be performed in the presence of infected ascites and may precipitate pulmonary oedema, bleeding from oesophageal varices, or disseminated intravascular coagulation.

Despite satisfactory control of ascites, the prognosis is poor with 50% of patients dying within 6 months, 75% within 1 year and 90% within 5 years.

Coagulation Defects

The liver manufactures prothrombin, fibrinogen, factors V, VII, IX and X. Although coagulation disturbances are common in liver failure, spontaneous bleeding is not a major problem and abnormalities can be improved by giving parenteral vitamin K. However, if bleeding does occur (more common in acute hepatic necrosis, see below), fresh frozen plasma should be given, together with platelets to correct any significant thrombocytopaenia ($<90 \times 10^9/\ell$).

Infection

The liver synthesizes alpha and beta globulins, and the Kupffer cells remove foreign material. In liver disease, the reduced globulins and bypassing of Kupffer cells, increase susceptibility to infection, particularly septicaemia or infection of ascites. Infection should, therefore, be excluded in any patient with known liver disease presenting with sudden deterioration.

Acute versus Chronic Liver Failure

Liver failure may be acute and potentially reversible or chronic and irreversible. In the UK the former is most common and occurs when the normal liver is severely damaged by acute viral hepatitis or drugs and when acute illness causes deterioration of chronic liver disease. The clinical features associated with these different types of liver failure are similar, with a few, important exceptions. Patients with acute hepatic necrosis are liable to become hypoglycaemic (*See Table 13*) while patients with underlying chronic liver disease develop hyperglycaemia. Bleeding is a greater problem in acute hepatic necrosis and several factors may be important. The liver is an important site of synthesis of clotting factors particularly the vitamin K dependent ones. As their half lives are short, coagulation deficiencies occur quickly. This is aggravated by reduced hepatic clearance of activated clotting factors and activation of the fibrinolytic system, secondary to disseminated intravascular coagulation. Chronic liver failure usually manifests as intractable hepatic encephalopathy and the usual measures to correct encephalopathy may not produce significant improvement. Since hepatic encephalopathy, is partly due to defective dopaminergic neurotransmission, levodopa and bromocriptine have been tried. The use of levodopa is limited by its gastrointestinal and neuropsychiatric side effects. However, bromocriptine, a specific dopamine receptor agonist (in doses up to 15 mg/day) has been reported to be of value to some patients.

Assessment of Pancreatic Function

The position of the pancreas in the retroperitoneal space has made non-surgical evaluation of this organ extremely difficult. In recent years, however, a number of techniques have been developed which enable definition of the anatomy and secretory function of the pancreas. Pancreatic disease may be classified as inflammatory, neoplastic, traumatic or genetic.

1. Inflammatory:	Acute and acute relapsing pancreatitis
	Chronic and chronic relapsing pancreatitis
2. Neoplastic:	Ductal
	Parenchymal
	Islet Cell
3. Traumatic:	Non-penetrating
	Penetrating
4. Genetic:	Cystic fibrosis
	Hereditary pancreatitis

In many of these disorders studies of pancreatic structure as well as secretory function are required to provide a definitive pathological diagnosis.

Exocrine Secretion

Faecal Studies

An estimation of the fat content of a 72 hour faecal collection provides an accurate diagnosis of fat malabsorption. Unfortunately, this test does not distinguish the cause of steatorrhoea although a very high fat output is suggestive of pancreatic insufficiency. Furthermore, the presence of steatorrhoea is not a sensitive indicator of pancreatic function and enzyme output is usually less than 10% of normal before fat absorption is significantly reduced. Measurements of faecal trypsin or chymotrypsin are also insensitive and of little diagnostic value.

Serum Enzyme Estimations

Measurement of serum and urinary amylase or lipase are extremely useful in diagnosing acute, acute relapsing and chronic relapsing pancreatitis. However, the magnitude of amylase elevation is not necessarily correlated with the severity of pancreatic damage and modest elevations of serum amylase may occur in other abdominal emergencies such as perforated peptic ulcer, gall bladder disease and intestinal ischaemia. The value of these tests in diagnosing other types of pancreatic disease, in particular chronic pancreatitis, remains in doubt. A marked rise in serum amylase or lipase after stimulation with secretin and/or pancreozymin has been used to indicate early pancreatic insufficiency. However, recent studies have shown that this test is neither sensitive nor specific.

Duodenal Intubation Studies

One of the most widely used tests of pancreatic function is the Lundh test, which has a sensitivity of around 80% and specificity of 90%. This involves intubation of the duodenum and estimation of duodenal enzyme activity, before and after stimulation with a meal. This investigation has been found to be abnormal in 90% of patients with chronic pancreatitis and 79% with pancreatic carcinoma. Although it is a simple, physiological and inexpensive test the results may be difficult to interpret after gastroduodenal surgery and when mucosal disease (e.g. Coeliac disease) impairs cholecystokinin and secretin release. Measurement of duodenal volume, enzyme and bicarbonate output after parenteral secretin or secretin plus cholecystokinin, has also been used to assess pancreatic function. In a recent survey of over 2000 patients, false positive results were found in 8% of healthy subjects and false negative results in 6% of patients. Although cannulation of the pancreatic duct at ERCP provides pure pancreatic juice, this investigation is technically very difficult and is currently of little value except for providing cytology samples during routine pancreatography *(see below)*.

Tubeless Tests of Pancreatic Exocrine Output

Hydrolysis of a synthetic tripeptide, N-benzoyl-L-tyrosyl-p amino-benzoic acid (NBT-PABA) has provided a simple and non-invasive test of pancreatic function. This compound is digested by chymotrypsin in the duodenum releasing PABA which is subsequently absorbed and excreted in the urine. After oral administration of a mixture of NBT-PABA and radio-labelled free PABA, urine is collected for 6–9 hours and the ratio of unlabelled to labelled PABA provides an estimation of pancreatic enzyme output. This test is abnormal in over 85% of patients with chronic pancreatitis and has a sensitivity of 75% and specificity of 95%. It is thus a useful screening procedure for pancreatic disease. The investigation is, however, expensive and abnormal results may occur in patients with renal insufficiency, abnormal hepatic function and if prunes, cranberries, sulphonylureas and sulphonamides are consumed during the test period.

Some recent studies suggest that the Triolein breath test may be adapted to assess pancreatic function. This test relies on the generation and absorption of ^{14}C labelled carbon dioxide, released when malabsorbed triolein is hydrolysed by colonic bacteria. A repeat test using pancreatic enzyme supplements has been shown to clearly distinguish between pancreatic insufficiency and mucosal disease causing steatorrhoea. However, these are preliminary studies and further data is required to confirm its clinical value.

Pancreatic Structure

Abdominal X-rays

Some useful information about the pancreas can be obtained from plain abdominal radiographs. Calcification occurs in both chronic idiopathic and alcoholic pancreatitis, while in acute pancreatitis, dilatation of small bowel loops ('sentinel sign') or abnormal gas patterns in the transverse colon ('colon cut-off sign') may be present. Abnormalities of pancreatic structure may also modify adjacent organs, such as the stomach and duodenum. The stomach may be displaced by a mass in the pancreatic head while masses in the body and tail may indent the duodenojejunal flexure. Deformities of the duodenum, caused by chronic pancreatitis and carcinoma, may be demonstrated by hypotonic duodenography but this procedure has been largely superceded by the scanning techniques discussed below. Carcinoma, at a late stage, produces filling defects in the duodenum and the 'inverted 3 sign of Frostberg'.

Radionuclide Scanning

Systemic administration of ^{75}Se-selenomethionine results in accumulation in those areas with active amino acid uptake, such as pancreas, liver and intestine. Clear visualization of the whole pancreas is useful in that it implies normal structure and function in over 95% of cases. However non-visualization of part or all of the organ may be due to intrinsic disease or variation in the positioning of the gland. The high false positive rate encountered (18%) severely limits the value of this test.

Ultrasound and Computerized Axial Tomography

Ultrasound scanning of the abdomen permits visualization of the pancreas in 80% of the patient population and has a specificity of 90% despite a low sensitivity (50%). Repeat examination after appropriate bowel preparation may enable imaging in a further 10%. In a study comparing ultrasound with barium meal, angiography and isotopic scanning, ultrasound proved to be the most accurate in diagnosing pancreatic disease. In acute pancreatitis, ultrasonography demonstrates uniform enlargement and a reduction in the echogenicity of the gland. In chronic pancreatitis echogenicity is enhanced and may be associated with calcification. Carcinoma of the pancreas produces a picture similar to acute pancreatitis except that the abnormality is more localized and may be associated with local spread, metastases or biliary obstruction. Ultrasonically guided biopsy of the pancreas may provide histological confirmation of the diagnosis. Ultrasonography may also detect the complications of pancreatitis, such as pseudocyst and abscess, and be used to assess the progress and resolution of such lesions.

Visualization of the normal pancreas by CT scanning depends to some extent on the presence of retroperitoneal fat planes that create significant contrast. The organ may be adequately outlined in 90% of normal subjects, but difficulties usually arise in very thin or cachectic patients. Abnormalities on the CT scan are observed in around 60–70% of patients with pancreatitis. In acute pancreatitis the gland may be diffusely swollen due to oedema, irregular in outline and of heterogeneous density. Complications of acute pancreatitis, such as pseudocyst, abscess and retroperitoneal extension of inflammation may also be demonstrated. The main diagnostic features of chronic pancreatitis are duct calculi, dilatation of the main duct and paraductal cysts. Pancreatic neoplasms may be identified in around 85% of patients but the majority are unresectable at that stage. CT scans of the pancreas are particularly useful in obese patients and in others not visualized by ultrasonography, but the cost of the procedure and its limited availability has restricted its use.

Endoscopic Retrograde Pancreatography

Endoscopic cannulation of the papilla of Vater was first described in 1968 and became widely used in the 1970's. With moderate experience (100 cases), most endoscopists quote a success rate of 85% for pancreatography and this investigation has a sensitivity of 80% and specificity of 65%. Complications develop in 2 – 3% of patients and the mortality rate is approximately 1 – 2/1000. Up to 83% of patients with chronic pancreatitis and 90% of those with pancreatic cancer may be correctly diagnosed at ERCP. Collection of pancreatic juice after secretin stimulation may add to the diagnostic yield, if abnormal cells are detected.

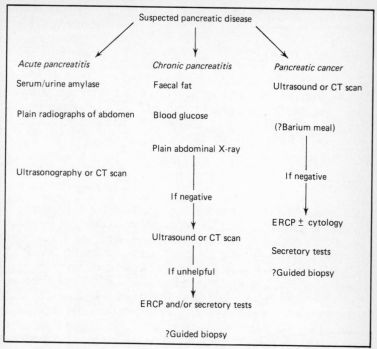

Figure 7 Diagnosis of pancreatic disease

'Which' Test

In patients with suspected acute pancreatitis, with or without complications, estimation of serum and urinary amylase together with ultrasonography should provide a diagnosis in most cases. In chronic pancreatitis, the diagnosis may be derived from faecal fat measurements, blood glucose profile and plain abdominal radiographs. If these investigations are unhelpful, ultrasonography plus secretory tests will detect at least 90% of cases. Ultrasound or CT scanning will diagnose pancreatic cancer in over 80% of cases and this yield is further increased if ERCP or secretory tests are performed.

Investigation of Diarrhoea

Diarrhoea is a very common disorder and one of the most frequent causes of industrial absenteeism from ill health in Britain. It can be caused by a wide variety of conditions and through a number of mechanisms, such as reduced absorption, active secretion, abnormalities of motility and altered permeability. Fortunately in most cases a diagnosis is made relatively easily following a clinical history and a few simple investigations.

History

Often the information obtained from a careful clinical history pinpoints the diagnosis or indicates the most appropriate investigations. It is important to take note of the onset, duration and severity of the diarrhoea and any associated symptoms. It is usually possible to identify whether the small intestine or large bowel is the source of diarrhoea. Small bowel diarrhoea usually has features of steatorrhoea (i.e. pale, greasy, offensive, bulky with a tendency to float), the volume is large and any associated pain tends to be peri-umbilical or situated in the right iliac fossa. Large bowel disorders tend to cause smaller volume stools as the diseased colon, being less tolerant of distension, will evacuate contents sooner than usual. Any associated pain tends to be lower abdominal or situated in either iliac fossa and tenesmus may be present. Blood and mucus in the stool also suggests large bowel disease. The pattern of diarrhoea may be helpful, for instance, alternating constipation and diarrhoea suggests irritable bowel syndrome while nocturnal diarrhoea suggests autonomic neuropathy due to diabetes or amyloidosis. Other systemic features may be of value. Weight loss or skin, joint and eye problems may all be associated with inflammatory bowel disease, peripheral neuropathy with amyloidosis and flushing with the carcinoid syndrome. A previous history of anal fistula, fissure or abscess may indicate Crohn's disease.

A family history, evidence of recent travel and documentation of drug intake are all essential. Drug induced diarrhoea is often overlooked and many common drugs such as antacids, cimetidine, digoxin, methyldopa and thiazide diuretics may be responsible for loose stools.

Examination

Clinical examination may reveal diagnostic pointers and should always include a digital rectal examination. Spurious diarrhoea due to severe constipation is not uncommon, especially in hospital practice and can easily be excluded by finding an empty rectum. The nutritional state of the patient may reflect the severity and source of the diarrhoea; signs of fat soluble vitamin deficiency (e.g. bruising) favouring small bowel disease. Anaemia, pigmentation, clubbing and skin, joint or eye signs should all be looked for. The presence of an abdominal mass suggests Crohn's disease, lymphoma or malignancy.

Investigations

From the above information the most appropriate investigations can be planned. Large bowel diarrhoea is investigated by stool cultures, sigmoidoscopy, barium enema and colonoscopy. Small bowel diarrhoea may require blood vitamin and haematinic levels, 3 day faecal fat collection, barium follow-through and jejunal biopsy. Further, more specialized, tests are usually held in reserve unless specifically indicated by the clinical features.

Stool Cultures

Fresh specimens should always be used for microscopy and culture as some organisms are temperature sensitive (e.g. amoebae) and only survive a short time in faeces. The bacteriology laboratory should be asked specifically to detect less common faecal pathogens like *Campylobacter* and *Clostridium difficile*. Repeated samples should be sent as the accuracy of diagnosis in some infestations increases if several specimens are examined (e.g. Giardiasis).

Sigmoidoscopy

Rigid sigmoidoscopy is easily and quickly performed on an unprepared patient and is an essential part of colonic investigations. Cleansing enemas should be avoided initially as they cause mucosal changes which may be misinterpreted as inflammation. Subsequently fibreoptic sigmoidoscopy, which requires prior preparation by a disposable phosphate enema, may allow visualization and biopsy of the left colon to the splenic flexure. The fine mucosal detail seen at fibreoptic examination enables the identification of vascular malformations and aphthous ulcers (seen in early Crohn's disease). Biopsy of a normal looking rectal mucosa in a patient with diarrhoea may reveal granulomata, thus confirming a diagnosis of Crohn's disease.

Barium Enema

A barium enema examination is only as good as the bowel preparation beforehand and to obtain good views of all areas this needs to be very thorough. Areas of difficulty for the radiologists are the caecum, sigmoid colon (especially when affected by diverticular disease) and the flexures. Double reading of X-rays improves diagnostic accuracy and it is important that films are looked at by two observers.

Colonoscopy

Colonoscopy is a second line investigation and is complementary to barium enema. It is particularly helpful in elucidating the cause of X-ray negative rectal bleeding or clarifying abnormalities seen on barium enema. The extent of inflammatory bowel disease can be accurately assessed and the terminal ileum inspected. Biopsy material can be obtained and this is especially helpful in assessing the degree of dysplasia in chronic ulcerative colitis.

Barium follow-through

An adequate barium examination must include views of all areas of the small bowel, in particular the terminal ileum. If the terminal ileum is not well shown the examination should be repeated or alternative arrangements made to visualize (e.g. colonoscopy, which would avoid further radiation exposure for the patient). Some authorities believe that the small bowel enema (where barium is introduced directly into the small bowel via a duodenal tube, avoiding dilution of the barium by stomach contents) is more accurate than a standard small bowel follow-through.

Jejunal Biopsy

A variety of methods are available to obtain biopsy samples of small bowel. Crosby and Watson capsules are the most frequently used instruments, but provide only a single specimen and occasionally contain no sample at all when removed. Multiple suction biopsies, although more difficult to obtain, provide a number of specimens and the biopsies are recovered before the sampling tube is removed. Endoscopic biopsies of the duodenum are useful, especially in patients in whom other techniques have failed. Some authorities consider endoscopic duodenal biopsies to be as accurate as formal jejunal biopsies in the diagnosis of coeliac disease. These may show evidence of Crohn's disease, intestinal lymphangiectasia or Whipple's disease. Jejunal aspiration can be performed at the same time as biopsy and is useful in the diagnosis of giardiasis or bacterial overgrowth.

Breath Tests

A variety of breath tests are available for the diagnosis of bacterial overgrowth of the small bowel. A number of pitfalls must be avoided if the test is to be reliable. Patients should not receive antibiotic therapy for 2 weeks prior to the test and other isotope tests must be deferred for a reasonable time before and after a radio-labelled breath test. Interpretation of breath tests is difficult at times and this is covered in detail elsewhere (*see* p. 113).

Therapeutic Trials

On occasions the responses to various drugs are used as diagnostic tests. Corticosteroids promote intestinal absorption by stimulating Na^+/K^+ activated ATPase in the mucosa and will improve many types of diarrhoea. The response to steroids cannot, therefore, be used as a diagnostic test for inflammatory bowel disease. On the other hand, bile salt induced diarrhoea may be difficult to confirm and a trial of cholestyramine may provide useful, indirect evidence of its presence. Likewise, with bacterial overgrowth, a trial of antibiotics may be justified in patients with suggestive features.

Investigation of persistent watery diarrhoea

On occasions the cause of diarrhoea is not established by the above investigations. At this stage admission to hospital may be useful, since it allows documentation of diarrhoea as well as enabling further investigation. The abrupt cessation of diarrhoea, in a patient admitted for investigation, suggests a functional disturbance (e.g. irritable bowel syndrome). Other easily overlooked causes of diarrhoea should be considered e.g. drug induced, thyrotoxicosis and internal fistulae. All tests and X-rays should be reviewed, paying particular attention to whether adequate views have been obtained of important areas. The possibility of laxative abuse should also be considered (see p. 50).

Osmotic and Secretory Diarrhoea

Diarrhoea can be divided into two major types. Osmotic diarrhoea, due to malabsorption of or ingestion of non-absorbable, osmotically-active solutes, rarely results in stool weight in excess of 400–500 g/day (normal stool weight on Western diet, approximately 200 g/day) and ceases (or is markedly reduced) by fasting for 24 – 48 hours. The stools often have a low pH (4–5). If the stools are sufficiently watery, faecal electrolytes and osmolality can be measured. The major cations are Na^+ and K^+ and these are balanced by equal concentrations of anions, the sum of $Na^+ + K^+$ in mmol/ℓ multiplied by 2 (to allow for anions) being approximately equal to stool osmolality in mOsm/kg. If stool osmolality is significantly greater than the sum of the ions measured, some osmotically active solute must be present to account for the ionic gap (e.g. lactose or magnesium). If an osmotic type of diarrhoea is confirmed, disaccharidase deficiency, osmotic purgative abuse, glucose/galactose malabsorption and less common malabsorption syndromes should be considered.

Secretory diarrhoea is characterized by large stool volumes (usually $> 1\ell$/day) and continues unabated during fasting. The exception to this rule is bile salt induced diarrhoea, which is reduced by fasting, since bile salts remain in the gall bladder. In secretory diarrhoea there is no ionic gap between measured stool electrolytes and faecal osmolality. Acute enteric infections cause secretory diarrhoea, but this is self-limiting and rarely causes a problem with diagnosis. In chronic secretory diarrhoea, purgative abuse and hormone producing tumours should be considered (see Table 14). Appropriate blood samples, collected from a fasting patient and stored correctly, should be sent for gut hormone analysis. It is advisable to send several specimens as hormone secretion may be intermittent. Investigations for laxative abuse should include: stool magnesium concentration, acidification of the urine (which turns pink in the presence of phenolphthalein) and tests for the presence of senna in stools and urine. A locker or hand-bag search may be necessary to confirm the diagnosis.

Conclusion

The cause of most diarrhoeal illness may be established from the clinical manifestations and simple investigations. An orderly approach, insisting on the accurate performance and interpretation of diagnostic tests, will yield dividends. More difficult cases benefit from in-patient observation and investigation.

Table 14: Hormonal causes of secretory diarrhoea

Condition	Agent responsible
Pancreatic cholera	Vasoactive intestinal polypeptide (VIP)
Zollinger–Ellison Syndrome	Gastrin
Carcinoid Syndrome	5-Hydroxytryptamine
Medullary carcinoma of thyroid	Calcitonin/prostaglandins
Ganglioneuroma	VIP

The Diagnosis and Management of Crohn's Disease

Introduction

Crohn's disease is an inflammatory condition, of unknown aetiology, affecting any part of the gastrointestinal tract. It has a wide distribution in the Western world; the incidence in the UK being 2–4/100 000 with a male to female ratio of 2:3. Patients may present at any age, with peak incidence in the third decade.

A variety of micro-organisms have been postulated as potential aetiological agents, as have diets high in refined sugars and low in dietary fibre. However clear evidence to support these hypotheses is lacking.

Disease Pattern

Site

The ileal and caecal regions are the commonest areas grossly involved (80%). Nearly 60% of patients have disease confined to the colon and the incidence of this type is rising faster than the other forms. Ten to fifteen per cent of patients have duodenal and jejunal disease. Areas apparently uninvolved may be functionally abnormal. The younger age groups are more likely to have small bowel involvement and the elderly, colonic disease.

Symptoms

The major symptoms are diarrhoea, abdominal pain and weight loss (50–90% of patients). Less commonly, rectal bleeding (40%), anal lesions (30–80%), fever (30%) and fistula (10%), occur. The abdominal pain may be due to active inflammation, abscess formation or obstruction and often more than one of these factors may be involved. The diarrhoea may be caused by active disease, past surgery (short bowel or post iliectomy *see* p. 166) or associated infections e.g. *Clostridium difficile*. About 30% of patients have an unremitting course despite therapy, while the remainder have intermittent relapses.

Extra-intestinal manifestations *(Table 15)*

These are more likely to occur in patients with colonic or ileocolonic disease. Twenty-five per cent of patients have at least one manifestation, with arthritis (19%) being the commonest feature. The presence of one manifestation increases the risk of developing another.

Complications

The common intestinal complications are abscesses, stricture formation leading to intestinal obstruction (particularly in the small bowel) and fistulae to other loops of bowel or adjacent organs (like bladder and vagina) and to the skin or surgical wounds. Patients who have had ileal surgery are at increased risk of developing gallstones and oxalate renal stones. In patients with ileostomies,

Table 15: Extra intestinal manifestations of Crohn's Disease

Type	Comment
Arthritis	
1. Peripheral synovitis	Non-erosive
2. Sacroiliitis ± spondylitis	Unrelated to disease activity
Skin	
1. Pyoderma gangrenosum	
2. Erythema nodosum	
3. Aphthous ulcers	6–10% of patients
4. Lichenoid	?Related to sulphasalazine
5. Malnutrition	Pellagra etc
6. Psoriasis	10% patients (?HLA related)
Eye	
1. Conjunctivitis	
2. Episcleritis	
3. Iritis	
Hepato-biliary	
1. Pericholangitis and Sclerosing Cholangitis	
2. Fatty liver	

sodium and water losses from the stoma can reduce urinary output and increase the incidence of uric acid stones. Ileo-caecal disease can cause ureteric compression leading to unilateral, obstructive hydronephrosis. There is an increased risk of developing gastro-intestinal malignancy in Crohn's disease (up to 10 times the normal population) and 37% of these occur in bypassed loops.

Diagnosis and Assessment

Diagnosis depends on the recognition of a pattern of clinical, radiological, endoscopic or histological features. The mean time from onset of symptoms to diagnosis is 3 years. Crohn's disease must be distinguished from an acute ileitis caused by Yersinia or Campylobacter infections since these rarely lead to chronic disease. Tuberculosis involves the ileo-caecal region but is rarely seen in the non-immigrant population (*see* p. 74). Ulcerative colitis is the major differential diagnosis when there is only colonic involvement with Crohn's disease. Histology, radiology and endoscopy can usually distinguish between the two conditions (*see* p. 192).

Pathology

The bowel is often segmentally involved (skip lesions) and there is relative sparing of the rectum (unlike colitis). The earliest lesions are aphthoid-like ulcers with normal intervening mucosa. More active disease leads to deep ulceration, fissuring, thickening and fibrosis of the bowel wall due to transmural inflammation. The inflammatory exudate is a mixture of acute and chronic cells, 50–70% of patients having non-caseating granulomata.

Haematology/Biochemistry

Blood loss, from active disease, malabsorption or inadequate intake of haematinics, may lead to iron or folate deficiency. Terminal ileal disease and resection can result in vitamin B_{12} deficiency. Plasma ESR is raised predominantly in colonic disease whilst upper intestinal disease leads to low plasma albumin, calcium, zinc, magnesium and other trace elements. The serum albumin may be low because of poor intake, malabsorption, protein losing enteropathy or inadequate synthesis secondary to sepsis and active disease. Fat malabsorption, from extensive disease, can result in decreased absorption of fat soluble vitamins A, D and K. Electrolyte abnormalities may occur in severe diarrhoea, particularly in those patients with ileostomies. Acute phase proteins, especially orosomucoids, are said by some authorities to be the most sensitive indicator of disease activity.

Radiology/Endoscopy

Radiology of the small and large bowel is helpful in delineating involved areas of bowel and may detect abscesses, fistulae or strictures. Sigmoidoscopy may reveal rectal disease and biopsies obtained may show granulomata. In patients with a normal appearing mucosa, biopsy is worthwhile since granulomata may be detected. Colonoscopy can view the entire colon and often the terminal ileum and provides an opportunity for histological diagnosis in those with normal radiology and sigmoidoscopy. In early Crohn's disease, colonoscopy will pick up typical aphthoid ulcers with intervening normal mucosa. A recent advance is radio-isotope imaging using labelled white blood cells. When re-injected into the patient these can be detected in areas of acute inflammation and abscesses.

Nutrition

A nutritional assessment (*see* p. 195) can reveal primary deficiencies and those secondary to small bowel disease or resection. Fifty per cent of patients have anorexia and their protein/calorie intake is often low. This may also be true for fibre, zinc and vitamin C intake (many patients find that fibre and vitamin C containing foods can exacerbate symptoms).

Management

Symptomatic

The anti-diarrhoeal opiates decrease intestinal transit and may increase fluid and electrolyte absorption. Codeine phosphate is cheap and effective, but loperamide is often preferred because it is little absorbed (allowing large doses to be administered) and increases anal sphincter tone (often reduced in these patients). In acute Crohn's colitis however there is a slight risk of opiates precipitating colonic dilatation. Cholestyramine may be helpful in choleric diarrhoea (*see* p. 84) but exacerbates steatorrhoea. There is widespread belief that bed rest in hospital provides symptomatic relief during a relapse.

Nutrition

Nutritional deficiencies need to be corrected and if tolerated, a high protein diet with appropriate supplements is ideal. Evidence, from controlled trials, that diet therapy can induce remissions or reduce disease activity is scanty. Elemental diets tend to be unpalatable and monotonous with few patients complying for any length of time. If steatorrhoea, hypolactasia or strictures are present a low fat, lactose free or low residue diet is required. If there is no contra-indication, a high fibre diet may be helpful in maintaining remission. Parenteral nutrition may be needed to correct deficiencies prior to surgery and in severely ill patients, particularly those with fistulae.

Specific Drugs

Corticosteroids are helpful in controlling active disease. Long term treatment has not been shown to prevent relapses or reduce complications but 10–15% of patients require low dose (up to 15 mg prednisolone/day) therapy to remain in remission. Acute severe relapses should be treated by parenteral steroids. The adverse effects of corticosteroids are dose dependent and since Crohn's patients may malabsorb prednisolone steroid complications develop at a higher dose than in patients with normal gut function. Sulphasalazine is beneficial in active Crohn's disease, particularly the colonic form. Small bowel disease may require a higher dose than usual (4–6g/day) but the benefit of sulphasalazine in quiescent, unremitting disease or after surgery is uncertain. Azathioprine and 6-mercaptopurine are used in patients with persisting disease and fistulae and have a steroid lowering effect. The risk of marrow suppression with these drugs has limited their use in this country. Metronidazole is helpful in perianal disease (*see* p. 122), fistulae and some abscesses while a recent trial suggests it may be as effective as sulphasalazine in patients with moderately active small bowel disease.

Surgery

Three quarters of patients require surgery for relief of obstruction, drainage of abscesses, resection of fistulae or removal of diseased bowel, unresponsive to medical therapy. Less common indications include toxic dilatation or uncontrolled haemorrhage. Resections should be limited to the segment(s) responsible for symptoms and radical excisions avoided. This is because surgery does not affect long term prognosis; relapse rate after surgery being nearly 100%. Multiple resections, if extensive, may also cause the short-bowel syndrome.

Prognosis

Although the mortality rate in Crohn's disease is twice that expected from a matched control population, long term studies suggest that 80% of patients will be leading normal lives, free of all therapy, 10–15 years after diagnosis.

The Assessment and Management of Nutritional Deficiencies

Assessment

Nutritional status can be estimated from a number of different parameters:

1. Dietary history
2. Clinical history and examination
3. Anthropometry
4. Biochemical tests

1. Diet

A careful dietary history is an essential baseline for nutritional assessment and helps distinguish dietary from pathological causes of an observed deficiency (e.g. folic acid). The patient's diet is compared to tables of 'Recommended Daily Intakes' for calories, protein, minerals, vitamins and trace elements. Although this is an imprecise method, if intake is adequate then deficiency is due to malabsorption or increased losses. Poor dietary intake may be due to economic, social or medical reasons. Non-gastrointestinal lesions like chronic obstructive airways disease, uraemia and congestive cardiac failure are all associated with malnutrition.

Optimal weight values are obtained from life insurance statistics. Weight (Wt) and height (H) are correlated to the body mass index (Mass index $= \dfrac{\text{Wt. kg}}{H^2.\,\text{cms}}$) and this ratio appears the best relation with body fat.

2. Clinical History and Examination

In patients with a clear cut history of gastrointestinal disease with steatorrhoea, nutritional deficiencies should be anticipated. As with other general medical conditions, gastrointestinal disease (e.g. peptic ulcer pain related to food intake) may result in diminished intake, as well as causing malabsorption or increased loss. Certain nutritional disorders (e.g. Scurvy) can be detected clinically, but this usually reflects moderate or severe deficiency (*see Table 16*). Milder deficiency states require further investigation.

Table 16

Physical Sign	Significance
Ecchymoses	Vitamin K deficiency
Petechial haemorrhage, Gut haemorrhage	Vitamin C deficiency
Chvostek's sign	↓ Calcium, magnesium, vitamin D
Pallor, Stomatitis	↓ Haematinics
Fissured erythematous tongue	↓ Niacin/thiamine
Eczematous pigmentation	↓ Niacin
Erythematous tongue + cheilosis	↓ Riboflavin
Proximal myopathy/tender bones	↓ Vitamin D
↓ Taste and hair with rough skin	Zinc deficiency
Oedema	Low albumin
Rough, dry skin	↓ Free fatty acid/zinc
Night blindness	↓ Vitamin A

3. Anthropometry

A distinction is made between lean body mass and body fat, as it is the former that has the greater prognostic value. Total body fat can be estimated by measuring skin fold thickness. This is performed by applying a skin caliper over the left triceps midway between the acromial and olecranon processes. Greater accuracy is obtained if three further sites (biceps, subscapular and iliac) are also sampled. Mean triceps skin fold thickness in the female varies from 8 mm in infancy to 18 mm[2] as an adult, whilst in males it is 10 mm throughout life. The lower limit of normal is 4 mm in males and 60% of the mean for age-matched females.

In starvation or disease, muscle protein is a sensitive index of lean body mass. The most convenient estimation of muscle mass is obtained by measuring the total circumference of the upper arm and subtracting the triceps skin fold thickness from this value. (Muscle circumference = Total circumference − Triceps skin fold thickness). The mean adult value is 280 mm for males and females, with values below 220 mm indicating muscle wasting.

4. Biochemistry

The serum albumin is the simplest biochemical parameter of malnutrition and is of predictive value in determining the prognosis and response to surgical procedures. Other causes of hypo-albuminaemia, like liver or renal disease must be excluded. Albumin is rapidly synthesized but its distribution and elimination are less predictable. Short term fluctuation in nutrition may, therefore, be more easily assessed using serum transferrin (rises with iron deficiency), caeruloplasmin, thyroid binding globulin and pre albumin.

Estimations of haemoglobin, iron, calcium, magnesium, zinc, copper, folate, B_{12} and immunoglobulins provide an indirect assessment of nutritional status.

Management

The body's metabolic requirements differ in starvation and injury. In starvation, sodium and water retention occur and insulin production falls, leading to amino acids being mobilized from stores, such as muscle, and utilized for glucose or albumin synthesis. Metabolic rate drops rapidly and 24 hour urinary nitrogen losses fall to 2–4 g/24 hours. If starvation continues, fat is increasingly utilized as an energy source. After injury there is a rise in metabolic rate with relatively less fat and more protein being utilized as calorie sources. Such catabolic states also occur after major surgery and intra-abdominal surgery. Thus nitrogen and calorie requirements differ in catabolic and non-catabolic states. Healthy adults require 8–9 g of nitrogen per day and this may need to be increased to over 20 g per day in severely catabolic patients (6.7 g Nitrogen = 1 g protein). Nitrogen balance studies can assess the need for further protein and positive balance of 1–2 g of nitrogen per day is all that is required. With a more positive balance unutilized nitrogen spills over into the urine or faeces and is wasted. Failure to achieve a positive nitrogen balance may be due to an inadequate nitrogen input, inadequate calorie input to prevent nitrogen being used as a calorie source, or excessive nitrogen losses e.g. high fistula output.

Indication for nutritional support is clear if there is overt malnutrition. Starved patients can be nutritionally repleted in a short period of time while catabolic patients require resolution of their 'injuries' before nutrition is restored to normal. Besides protein and calories, these patients require adequate mineral, vitamin and trace elements. When the absorptive site of the gastrointestinal tract (duodenum and jejunum) is normal, enteral feeding should be attempted using whole or liquid foods. In many patients, a protein or calorie supplement may be all that is required (e.g. Ensure,

Nutrauxil, Complan). Although elemental diets contain pre-digested' food, these are unpalatable and the high osmolality may cause troublesome diarrhoea. Parenteral nutrition should be confined to patients who cannot tolerate oral feeding, have absent, diseased or non-functioning upper small bowel, or have high output intestinal fistulae. Total parenteral nutrition should be administered through a central venous line and maintained by a trained multi-disciplinary parenteral nutrition team. This will help reduce the incidence of catheter sepsis, the major complication of this treatment. When recovery from intestinal failure may be prolonged or inadequate, such parenteral nutrition may be continued in the patient's home.

Further Reading

Alexander-Williams, J. and Binder, H. J. (eds.) (1983). *Gastroenterology 3: Large Intestine*, (London: Butterworths)

Baron, J. H. and Moody, F. G. (eds.) (1981). *Gastroenterology 1: Foregut* (London: Butterworths)

Chadwick, V. S. and Phillips, S. F. (eds.) (1982). *Gastroenterology 2: Small Intestine*, (London: Butterworths)

Classen, M. and Schreiber, H. W. (eds.) (1983). Biliary tract disorders, *Clinics in Gastroenterology*, vol. 12.1 (London: W. B. Saunders Co)

Howat, H. T. and Sarles, W. B. (1979). *The Exocrine Pancreas* (London: W. B. Saunders Co)

Irving, M. H. and Beart, R. W. (eds.) (1983). *Surgery 3: Gastroenterological Surgery* (London: Butterworths)

Sherlock, S. (1981). *Diseases of the Liver and Biliary System* (Oxford: Blackwell Scientific Publications)

Sleisenger, M. H. (ed.) (1983). Malabsorption and Nutritional Support, *Clinics in Gastroenterology*, vol. 12.2 (London: W. B. Saunders Co)

Sleisenger, M. H. and Fordtran, J. S. (eds.) (1978). Gastrointestinal Disease, *Pathophysiology, Diagnosis and Management* (London: W. B. Saunders Co)

Wright, R. (ed.) (1980). Recent Advances in Gastrointestinal Pathology (London: W. B. Saunders & Co)

Wright, R., Alberti, K. G. M. M., Karran, S., Millward-Sadler, G. H. (eds.) (1979). Liver and Biliary Disease, *Pathophysiology, Diagnosis and Management* (London: W. B. Saunders Co)

Index of Cases

	Case Number	Discussion Pages
Oesophagus		
Achalasia	12	64–66
Oesophageal Stricture	59	152–153
Oesophageal varices	46	128–130
Oesophageal webs and rings	8	58–59
Oesophagitis	6	54–56
Stomach		
Drug-induced haemorrhage	33	102–104
Post-gastrectomy dumping	49	133–135
Stump carcinoma	34	104–106
Zollinger–Ellison Syndrome	5	53–54
Small intestine		
Angiodysplasia	10	60–62
Ascariasis	14	67–69
Autonomic neuropathy	13	66–67
Carcinoid syndrome	50	135–137
Coeliac disease	23	84–86
Crohn's disease	39	114–115
Gall stone obstruction	9	59–60
Ileocaecal tuberculosis	17	73–75
Intestinal ischaemia	47	130–131
Intestinal lymphangiectasia	45	126–128
Jejunal diverticulosis	38	111–114
Lactose intolerance	29	95–97
Lymphoma	35	106–107
Peutz–Jeghers Syndrome	4	51–53
Primary immune deficiency syndromes	40	115–117
Radiation enteritis	31	99–100
Scleroderma	58	151–152
Traveller's diarrhoea	42	119–121
Vipoma	30	97–98
Whipple's disease	55	145–146

Large intestine

Amoebic colitis	21	81–82
Bile salt induced diarrhoea	22	83–84
Caecal carcinoma	53	141–143
Crohn's colitis	7	57–58
Diverticular disease	15	70–71
Irritable bowel syndrome	25	87–89
Ischaemic colitis	20	79–80
Laxative abuse	3	50–51
Perianal Crohn's disease	43	121–123
Pneumatosis coli	54	144–145
Pseudomembranous colitis	2	48–50
Sigmoid volvulus	57	149–150
Solitary rectal ulcer	18	75–77
Ulcerative colitis	48	131–133
Ulcerative proctitis	51	137–139

Hepatobiliary

Alcoholic hepatitis	36	108–109
Cholangiocarcinoma	52	139–141
Drug-induced hepatocellular damage	44	123–125
Emphysematous cholecystitis	41	118–119
Gall stones	37	110–111
Gilbert's Syndrome	28	93–95
Haemochromatosis	27	91–93
Hepatic adenomas	24	86–87
Portal vein thrombosis	32	100–102
Primary biliary cirrhosis	19	77–78
Pyogenic liver abcess	1	47–48
Viral hepatitis	56	146–149
Wilson's disease	11	62–64

Pancreas

Carcinoma of pancreas	60	154–155
Chronic pancreatitis	16	72–73
Pancreatic atrophy	26	89–91

Case Presentations in Renal Medicine

R. A. Coward, MRCP
Research Fellow, Department of Renal Medicine, Manchester Royal Infirmary

C. D. Short, MRCP
Tutor in Medicine, Department of Renal Medicine, Manchester Royal Infirmary

N. P. Mallick, FRCP
Consultant Physician, Department of Renal Medicine, Manchester Royal Infirmary

1983   *192 pages*   *0 407 00232 4*   *Softcover*

This concise and informative book aims to involve the reader directly in the clinical analysis and the decision making about patients suffering from kidney disease.

The authors, based in a busy nephrological centre, present 58 carefully selected cases, followed by questions about diagnosis, investigation and management. For each case they provide a commentary which discusses the major issues arising from it and answers the questions posed. In this way the reader gains valuable experience in practical clinical thinking and absorbs information about renal medicine in a vivid and easily assimilable fashion.

Towards the end of the book, a section is devoted to explaining important and poorly understood topics, such as creatinine clearance, imaging in renal disease and continuous ambulatory peritoneal dialysis.

The result is an invaluable textbook aimed principally at those studying for higher professional qualifications in medicine. Students at an earlier stage in their clinical career will also profit from it, as indeed will all those with an interest and involvement in nephrology.

Case Presentations in Paediatrics

Vanda Joss, MRCP
Consultant Paediatrician, Milton Keynes Hospital

Stephen J. Rose, MRCP
Lecturer in Child Health, University of Aberdeen

1983   *265 pages*   *0 407 00234 0*   *Softcover*

Many higher professional examinations in medicine, for example those for the Membership of the various Royal Colleges of Physicians, require candidates to exercise their powers of clinical judgement in so-called 'grey' cases.

In this valuable book, Dr Joss and Dr Rose have compiled 77 such cases. Each case presentation is followed by questions, answers and a carefully reasoned discussion; there is also a guide to further reading for those who remain puzzled or who want to broaden their understanding.

Case Presentations in Paediatrics is an indispensable aid for all those taking higher professional examinations in paediatrics or general medicine. Students at an earlier stage in their clinical career will also profit from it.

After reading this book candidates will feel confident of avoiding even the most cunning traps that examiners can set, and be secure in the knowledge that they have advanced their general understanding of clinical paediatrics.

Case Presentations in Heart Disease

Alan Mackintosh, MA, MD, MRCP
Consultant Cardiologist, St James's University and Killingbeck Hospitals, Leeds

1985   *176 pages*   *0 407 00541 2*   *Softcover*

Medicine in books and in the real world do not always correlate. This book of 52 case presentations complements existing textbooks by putting heart disease firmly back into the hospital and GP's surgery. It reflects the normal medical process by starting with the symptoms and signs, and then explores the possible diagnosis and treatment. The patients are presented as they would appear in the GP's surgery, hospital clinic or ward. At the end of each case there are questions, and the second half of the book contains discussions and the answers.

The cases are representative of present-day cardiology, from emergencies to long-term illnesses. Common diseases are emphasized, but some rarities also appear. The author writes entertainingly, and his skillful and realistic description of cases provides ample opportunity for readers to exercise their clinical judgement.

Dr Mackintosh's book is intended primarily for those preparing for higher professional examinations such as the MRCP and the MRCGP. In addition senior clinical students and qualified physicians will find the book instructive and illuminating.

Available through all good booksellers or from the publishers

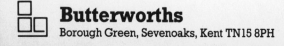

Butterworths
Borough Green, Sevenoaks, Kent TN15 8PH